The Yoga Zoo Adventure

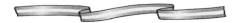

About the Author

Helen Purperhart is mother to Nina (age 12) and Carmel (age 5). She runs a yoga center called Jip and Jan in Almere, Holland, where she teaches a number of children's yoga workshops and trains prospective children's yoga teachers. Through her work, Helen aims to change the way teachers and parents see and interact with children.

Helen is the author of *The Yoga Adventure for Children* and *Yoga Exercises for Teens,* also published by Hunter House Publishers.

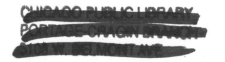

SmartFun Books from Hunter House

101 Music Games for Children by Jerry Storms

101 More Music Games for Children by Jerry Storms

101 Dance Games for Children by Paul Rooyackers

101 More Dance Games for Children by Paul Rooyackers

101 Drama Games for Children by Paul Rooyackers

101 More Drama Games for Children by Paul Rooyackers

101 Movement Games for Children by Huberta Wiertsema

101 Language Games for Children by Paul Rooyackers

101 Improv Games for Children by Bob Bedore

101 Life Skills Games for Children by Bernie Badegruber

101 More Life Skills Games for Children by Bernie Badegruber

101 Cool Pool Games for Children by Kim Rodomista

101 Family Vacation Games by Shando Varda

101 Relaxation Games for Children by Allison Bartl

101 Quick-Thinking Games + Riddles for Children by Allison Bartl

101 Pep-Up Games for Children by Allison Bartl

404 Deskside Activities for Energetic Kids by Barbara Davis, MA, MFA

Yoga Games for Children by Danielle Bersma and Marjoke Visscher

The Yoga Adventure for Children by Helen Purperhart

Yoga Exercises for Teens by Helen Purperhart

The Yoga Zoo Adventure by Helen Purperhart

Ordering

Trade bookstores in the U.S. and Canada please contact:

Publishers Group West
1700 Fourth St., Berkeley CA 94710
Phone: (800) 788-3123   Fax: (800) 351-5073

Hunter House books are available at bulk discounts for textbook course adoptions;
to qualifying community, health-care, and government organizations;
and for special promotions and fund-raising. For details please contact:

Special Sales Department
Hunter House Inc., PO Box 2914, Alameda CA 94501-0914
Phone: (510) 865-5282   Fax: (510) 865-4295
E-mail: ordering@hunterhouse.com

Individuals can order our books from most bookstores,
by calling **(800) 266-5592**, or from our website at
www.hunterhouse.com

The Yoga Zoo Adventure

Animal Poses and Games for Little Kids

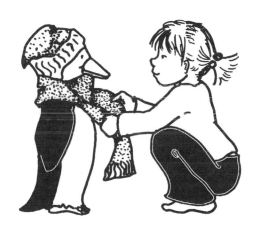

Helen Purperhart

Translated by Amina Marix Evans
Illustrated by Barbara van Amelsfort

A Hunter House SmartFun Book

Library of Congress Cataloging-in-Publication Data

Purperhart, Helen.
The yoga zoo adventure : animal poses and games for little kids
/ Helen Purperhart ; translated by Amina Marix Evans ; illustrated by
Barbara van Amelsfort. — 1st ed.
p. cm. — (SmartFun book)
ISBN-13: 978-0-89793-505-0 (pbk.)
ISBN-10: 0-89793-505-5 (pbk.)
ISBN-13: 978-0-89793-506-7 (spiral bound)
ISBN-10: 0-89793-506-3 (spiral bound)
1. Hatha yoga for children—Juvenile literature.
2. Animals—Juvenile literature.   I. Title.
RJ133.7.P87 2008
613.7'046083—dc22   2008004042

Project Credits

Cover Design: Jil Weil & Stefanie Gold
Illustrations: Barbara van Amelsfort
Book Production: John McKercher
Translator: Amina Marix Evans
Developmental and Copy Editor: Colleen Sell
Proofreader: Herman Leung
Acquisitions Editor: Jeanne Brondino
Editor: Alexandra Mummery

Senior Marketing Associate: Reina Santana
Publicity Assistant: Alexi Ueltzen
Rights Coordinator: Candace Groskreutz
Customer Service Manager:
   Christina Sverdrup
Order Fulfillment: Washul Lakdhon
Administrator: Theresa Nelson
Computer Support: Peter Eichelberger
Publisher: Kiran S. Rana

Printed and Bound by Bang Printing, Brainerd, Minnesota

Manufactured in the United States of America

9 8 7 6 5 4 3 2 1   First Edition   08 09 10 11 12

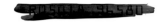

Contents

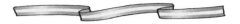

A detailed list of the games indicating appropriate group sizes begins on the next page.

*Please note that the illustrations in this book are all outline drawings.
The fact that the pages are white does not imply that the people all have white skin. This
book is for people of all races and ethnic identities.*

List **of** Games

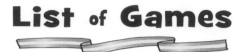

List of Stories

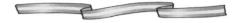

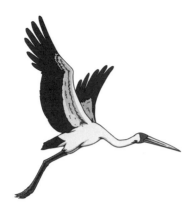

Dedication

I dedicate this book to all the conservationists
in the world who are working to protect animals
and to preserve their natural environment.

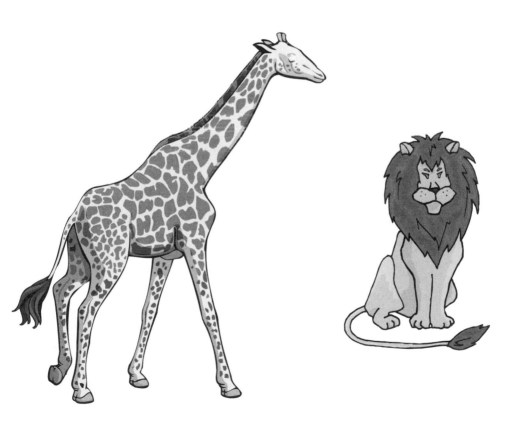

Important Note

The material in this book is intended to provide information about a safe, enjoyable exercise program for children. Every effort has been made to provide accurate and dependable information. The contents of this book have been compiled through professional research and in consultation with professionals. However, professionals have differing opinions, and some of the information may become outdated; therefore, the publisher, authors, and editors, as well as the professionals quoted in the book cannot be held responsible for any error, omission, or dated material. The authors and publisher assume no responsibility for any outcome of applying the information in this book. Follow the instructions closely. Note that children's bodies are fragile, so they should not be forced to assume any physical positions that cause them pain or discomfort. If you have questions concerning your exercise program or about the application of the information described in this book, consult a qualified yoga professional.

Foreword

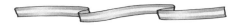

"Oaaaaahgrrrf." There is a strange sound coming from Helen Purperhart's yoga room. Whatever is she doing now?

I have been friends with Helen Purperhart for several years, and her approach to teaching yoga is very special. No matter when you visit her yoga studio, she is always researching, deepening her insight and learning the latest information about her profession. She approaches her work with great enthusiasm and always encourages others to work in their own way. Over the years, Helen has been a great source of inspiration for many students and teachers of yoga.

In *The Yoga Zoo Adventure*, Helen adds a dimension to yoga that many of us have forgotten: our basic animal nature, the innate connection between humans and animals. Through a series of exercises incorporated into fun games, children discover and emulate the movements that different animals make. How does it feel to be bigger or smaller than you are? Faster or slower? Stronger or weaker? These games not only open up an exciting new world for children, they are also enjoyable for adults and tell them much about their young charges.

Many of us have pets for the companionship they provide, but animals also have much to teach us. This book will help children and adults alike to look at animals in a different way—one that brings them closer to nature and gives them more insight into the animal kingdom. In learning about a variety of animals, we learn more about ourselves. By becoming closer with nature, we get closer to ourselves. The better we understand animals, the better we understand ourselves. Each animal speaks to us, if we would only learn how to listen. Animals can teach us how to survive or to adapt, how to be powerful or courageous. They show us many qualities that we can develop in ourselves. They help us to become more aware of our own powers and possibilities. Animals, like children, reawaken our sense of wonder and our belief in dreams and unending possibilities.

This philosophizing takes me back to the period when, as a small child, I had the opportunity to live in the jungle of Suriname for a few weeks. The overwhelming nights—signaled at 6:00 P.M. by the sound of a thousand crickets, by the flying fish that flew right into my face when we were fishing at night by lamplight, and by the rituals the Javanese performed with animals—are unforgettable experiences I carry with me still. Helen wrote this book for those who have not had the opportunity to experience nature in such a way. Many children today have few opportunities to celebrate and explore their place in the natural world with their bodies, minds, feelings, and spirits and with creativity and humor.

In *The Yoga Zoo Adventure*, Helen reveals her primitive side and shares it with everyone. The book's games, exercises, songs, and stories will carry children and their instructors away to the animal kingdom, where all will discover the magic of nature, movement, and play. I return now to the yoga room, fascinated to know which animal I might find there.

— Emeke Buitelaar, September 2006

About the Author

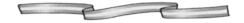

"This is it," thought Helen Purperhart during a yoga class for pregnant women she was taking thirteen years ago. Everything she had learned until then came together in that moment, inspiring her to become a yoga instructor. As she trained for her new career, Helen realized she wanted to teach yoga to kids, so she took a specialized course on yoga for children. There, she learned how yoga and movement games could help children to develop a better awareness of their bodies and improve their emotional as well as their physical well-being.

She believes that parents and teachers provide an important mirror for children; with kids, nothing beats a good role model. By the same token, a child is a mirror for the parent or teacher, projecting and enlarging those things in ourselves that we adults try to hide. Doing yoga with children, Helen believes, gives you the chance to rediscover and release your own inner child, to suspend inhibitions and to experience more pleasure, appreciation, enthusiasm, curiosity, trust, and joy. Most importantly, spending this type of quality time together with children helps them to build positive relationships while engaging in a fun and fitness-enhancing activity.

Acknowledgments

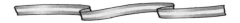

My thanks go first to my oldest friend, Sophie van der Zee, who has again helped me enormously with adapting the stories and exercises to suit young children. She also reminded me constantly of the need to use simple language in communicating the essence of yoga.

Loving thanks go to my best friend, Emeke Buitelaar, for writing the Foreword and for the beautiful adventures we have experienced together.

I am thankful to Marion Gravendaal, Sanna Maris, Leonieke de Wildt, and Elly de Wildt-Dienske for their feedback after reading the manuscript, to Veronique Veenendaal for her idea and poem for the exercise "Dance of the Night," to Barbara van Amelsfort for the cheery illustrations, and to Anneke Dijk for doing all the exercises together with me.

I also thank Halbo C. Kool and Arnold Lobel for inspiring me to write my updated versions of the animal fables.

Finally, I thank all those to whom I have taught children's yoga for their enthusiasm and support and for the joyful times we've shared.

When Children Play

Elephants *walk* on soft cushions,
Tigers *stalk* between the bushes,
Frogs *jump* into the pond,
Penguins *dive* into the hole in the ice,
Sharks *swim* in the ocean,
Apes *swing* from tree to tree,
Birds *fly* in the air,
Snakes *slither* over the ground,

But when children play, they can choose:

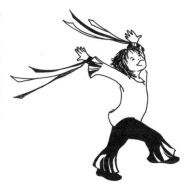

They *walk* and *trumpet,*
They *slither* and *roar,*
They *jump* and *quack*
They *dive* and *bray,*
They *swim silently,*
They *swing* and *laugh*
They *fly* and *flutter*
And *creep* around *hissing.*

— *Helen Purperhart*

Introduction

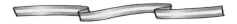

I still remember my youngest daughter's beautiful sense of wonder during a family outing to the zoo. It was her first conscious visit to the zoo, when she was old enough to observe and understand what she was experiencing. Carmel is very interested in animals, especially things that crawl, fly, and buzz. So we went through the zoo full of expectation. Carmel thought everything was wonderful. The monkeys were fun. Coming face-to-face with lions and tigers was exciting. The huge elephants and the giraffes with their unbelievably long necks were fascinating. She knew about bears, because she had a teddy of her own.

On the path in front of the lion's enclosure, Carmel found a tiny dead mouse, and instead of looking at the amazing lions, she and her older sister became totally absorbed in the mouse. Their excitement over the ordinary mouse was extraordinary, and we were all enlisted to gather twigs and leaves in order to give him a proper burial.

All in all, the day was a great success, and the children learned a lot. It was such a memorable experience that for months afterward if someone asked Carmel where she had been with Mum and Dad, she always said "to the zoo." Of course, if asked now what she'd seen there, she would likely say "a dead mouse and a teddy bear." The mouse was the highlight of the day for our daughters, even more interesting than all the other amazing and exotic animals they saw.

That delightful visit to the zoo sparked the idea for this book—a collection of animal-themed yoga exercises especially for young children, ages three to seven.

The Yoga Zoo Adventure begins with practical information for parents and teachers. This section explains what yoga is and its benefits to children. It also provides advice on how to structure and conduct the lessons.

The second part of the book is a guided tour through the zoo. It includes numerous yoga-based exercises—all played as games, many with songs and stories—in which children use their bodies and their imaginations to emulate the shapes and movements of various animals. The book's straightforward, step-by-step instructions make the exercises easy to teach and to learn, and the games, songs, and stories create a playful experience children are sure to enjoy.

Next, a collection of animal fables helps children to learn the underlying philosophies of yoga in a simple and lighthearted way.

The last section of the book provides information about zoos and the animals that live there. You can use this information as a reference to deepen your knowledge of the animals—all the better to answer the inevitable questions that will come from the children as they make this journey through the animal kingdom.

The main aim of *The Yoga Zoo Adventure* is to motivate teachers and parents to take a relaxed and playful approach toward yoga for children by integrating exercise with music, dance, storytelling, breathing, relaxation, and play. If this book prompts people to laugh, play, move, discover, and enjoy together, then it has achieved its purpose.

Guidelines for Parents and Teachers

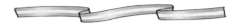

What Is Yoga?

Yoga existed in India for a couple of thousand years before we began counting time. The word yoga means "binding." Through the practice of yoga, you bind—or integrate—the physical, mental, and spiritual elements of your life. Yoga is the way to consciousness of the unity and connectedness of everything in the universe: people, animals, plants, earth, air, water. Yoga also means the search for the oneness, the truth, and the freedom that exists within us. The development of qualities such as courage and trust are preconditions for reaching this inner peace. Learning the art of relaxation is also of huge importance in this endeavor. Of course, no one can achieve this idealistic state of being with one hour of yoga a week. It takes time and effort, sometimes a lifetime of effort. However, yoga can help instill these qualities in children as well as adults, who can then find their own ways of mastering this in their daily lives.

In essence, yoga is concerned with stilling your thoughts, which begins with simple forms of self-discipline and self-control. These techniques for living more consciously and more healthily are described in ancient Indian texts, the most well-known of which is that of Patanjali, who set forth the *eightfold path* of yoga in the form of rules for living.

The Eightfold Path

The *first step* on the path of yoga covers the *five abstentions*, which involves abstaining from the "bad habits" of violence, lying, theft, gluttony, and greed.

The *second step* on the path of yoga takes the form of the *five precepts*. These grow out of the abstentions and involves acquiring five good habits: purity, contentment, self-discipline, self-directed learning, and devotion.

The way of yoga begins with improving and developing your physical body to its optimal point through various *yoga postures*. These exercises bring physical health, strength, and suppleness. They are the best-known elements of yoga and form the *third step* on the yogic path. Only when you have achieved a certain amount of mastery over your body can you achieve mastery of your mind—over how and what you think.

The *fourth step* on the yogic path is the practice of *breathing exercises*. These help with gaining control of your energy to bring more vitality.

The *fifth step* is the practice of *directing your attention* inward, independent of the senses. This helps to bring about emotional rest.

The *sixth step* is the practice of *focusing* on a specific point or image, such as a candle flame, flower, or mantra, in order to increase spiritual strength.

The *seventh step* is the practice of *meditation,* which helps to prevent disturbing thoughts from upsetting the concentration.

The *eighth step* on the eightfold path forms true knowledge, or *enlightenment*, a conscious awareness of one's unity with the universe and with God, unrestricted by judgment.

Today, yoga is practiced in both the East and the West, and there are many types of yoga, each of which interprets yoga in its own way. This book does not aim to give a complete picture of the classic yoga system and all its variations, but it does give a good idea of the basic life rules of yoga and how they can be applied to children's yoga. The main focal points of yoga for children are discovery, movement, and fantasy.

Why Yoga for Children?

Children's yoga has become very popular recently because it is a wonderful way for kids to move and to relax. Yoga's calming effect on children, even those who are very young, is particularly appealing to parents. Young children are bursting with energy and love moving about, so what could be better than discovering yoga through play?

This play-based approach to children's yoga—through fun and imaginative games, songs, exercises, and stories—incorporates all the essential components of yoga:

- relaxation
- breathing
- physical contact and massage
- attention and concentration
- stimulation of the senses

- physical consciousness and movement
- development of motor skills

Children's yoga is a voyage of discovery in which each child can develop at her or his own pace. Exercises and games aimed at coordination, motor skills, and suppleness improve and refine children's capabilities for movement and increase their body awareness. This, in turn, helps to create a link between their physical being and their emotions, thinking, social skills, and imagination. Working together and listening to each other stimulate empathy and the ability to express their feelings. They learn to take initiative and to accept the initiatives of others. By talking about all the things they have experienced, they give form to who they are and what they feel. Even those children who find it difficult to express how they feel and what they experience during the yoga class find that yoga makes them feel calmer and helps them to discover new things about themselves.

Playing with Nature

Children are intuitively aware that they are part of nature and the universe, and they are totally absorbed in the world around them. Their senses are wide open and their attention is constantly drawn to things outside themselves—images, sounds, colors, smells, tastes, and the tactile sensations of touching or being touched by something or someone. Children experience the world through their senses. They are acutely aware of the cool rain or the warm breeze on their faces; the squishy mud or soft grass beneath their feet; the silky fur of a kitten or the slimy skin of a frog on their fingertips. They are sensitive to the scents of flowers and damp earth; the sounds of birdsong and mooing cows; the colors and shapes of flowers, trees, and animals; and the tastes of sour, sweet, salty, and bitter.

The stimulation of the senses plays an important role in yoga lessons for children. When these lessons are fun games that are based on natural themes, children also learn about nature and about themselves. For example, in one exercise they might grow from small seeds into a strong tree and let their branches move in the wind, while drumming with their fingers on their body to simulate the feel and sound of rain.

Children respond to sensory stimuli with their entire being—not only with their emotions and words but also with their bodies. Yoga helps children to express themselves with posture, movement, and gestures, giving voice to ideas and feelings that might otherwise remain hidden.

Learning Through Play

Structured play is one of the most effective teaching methods for young children, and children can learn a variety of skills from yoga lessons that feature creative play. The movement not only improves physical fitness, it also helps kids to understand such spatial concepts as above, under, forward, behind, left, and right. Play makes excercise more engaging and fun, which in turn enhances the children's ability to focus and to channel their energy. Doing yoga games together with others—whether it be siblings, a group of kids, or a sole parent or instructor—helps kids to develop their interpersonal skills. All of the skills resulting from this type of structured play carry over to children's daily activities and will be needed in their adult lives.

Another aspect of playing that can be of great enjoyment and benefit to children is imagination. Most children transition smoothly between reality and fantasy, and by encouraging and guiding that process, you can turn a lesson into an exciting adventure. Using their imaginations allows children to explore the world around them as well as their own ideas and feelings without inhibition. It enables them to recreate experiences from their lives, providing a playful way for them to process those events and to prepare themselves for what is to come. It facilitates the development of creative thought, which is an important component of problem-solving. Imaginative play can also inspire a child to reach farther—to envision and work toward loftier goals than what might seem plausible or acceptable in the "real world."

Adults, too, can envision a situation in their minds and thus prepare themselves for it. This ability is largely a result of childhood games and the daydreams of later life. Teachers and parents who use their imaginations when teaching yoga to children and who enjoy engaging in imaginative play with children will inspire those children to let their fantasies run free.

How to Use This Book

The Games section of *The Yoga Zoo Adventure* contains several components:

- step-by-step written instructions for each exercise or activity

- illustrations of animals and of children at play
- a list of any props needed to play a specific game
- the words to each song or rhyme accompanying a game
- a running story that narrates the children's journey through the zoo

For most of the games, the instructions are written to be read by the parent or teacher out loud, word for word, to the children. These are printed in italics. For some games, the instructions are written as guidelines for the parent or teacher, who will need to use their own words to teach and guide the children through the games. Those instructions are in regular type.

The drawings are intended chiefly for visual interest. Some of them illustrate the exercises, and those should be used in conjunction with, not instead of, the written instructions. It is very important to carefully follow the written instructions.

The continuous story is scattered throughout the Games section of the book. It appears in the special font below and is set off by paw prints.

It is morning. Soon you will begin your zoo adventure, but first you must wake up.

The descriptions of the exercises should be seen as guides within which there is ample room for creativity. You can combine your own ideas with those in the book; you can also incorporate ideas that the children bring. The main thing is to use creativity when putting together your lesson.

Planning the Lesson

The intention of this book is to get children, parents, and teachers moving. It is not a textbook that children need to work through. Sometimes children are not able to do a particular exercise, in which case you could modify it or simply exclude it from the lesson. You can always come back to it later.

The exercises in this book are intended to offer new experiences that make use of the natural curiosity of small children. Some of the exercises are particularly well-suited for learning specific skills, but you can always do an exercise simply because it's fun!

Because most kids love animals, this book is based on a visit to the zoo, but there are countless other situations to which you could apply these exercises and games. You could pick out a number of exercises and put together your own adventure grouped around a different theme. You could use different stories, games, and songs.

You should feel free to use the games in whatever order and to tailor them to whatever theme suits your purpose and the children's abilities and interests.

Of course, you can do the exercises in the order suggested in the book and follow along with the zoo adventure. For example, you could plan lessons for a "zoo week," working on a part of the book each day. Small children learn a little more each day, and they enjoy it enormously when they recognize the animals the next time they come across them in a book or in real life. You could also do different animals or exercises, or simply change the sequence of the exercises.

Before you can plan the lesson, you will need to decide the theme of the lesson and select the games that fit your chosen theme. You will also need to decide whether and how to change any of the exercises, stories, and songs. Finally, you should gather any props you might need for the lesson.

Keep in mind that with very young children you will need to demonstrate a lot and talk a little. Kids of this age tend to have shorter attention spans and to learn better from example than from verbal instruction. This is especially true of preschoolers (3- to 5-year-olds).

A lesson might look something like this:

1. **Introduction**

    At the start of the lesson, tell the children what it will be about. Keep it short and simple, describing the nature of the activity in general terms. You can also mention aspects that will be included later in the lesson.

2. **Warm Up**

    For younger children, a playful warm-up exercise is a good start. For example, you could begin each lesson with the "Rise and Shine" games.

3. **Exercise and Play Time**

In this part of the lesson, you will guide the children in doing the games you've selected for your chosen theme. You can use whatever exercises, songs, stories, and props you've selected to enhance the lesson's playfulness. For example, if you follow the zoo adventure in this book, you could hang up pictures of the animals featured in the lesson or bring in toy animals to introduce them individually. The children can then respond to the picture or the toy.

4. **Cool Down**

The lesson can be concluded in various ways. You could do the "Settle Down" games in this book. Another option is to finish the lesson with an improvisation session in which each child demonstrates their own variation of an exercise from the lesson to the rest of the class. Other options include reading the children a story related to the theme or leading the children in a song related to the theme.

Starting the Lesson

Before you begin, choose a space where there is a minimum of distraction and plenty of space to move freely. This could be an empty classroom, a gym, a playroom, or a family room. At home, children can also choose their own space where they can go to quietly practice their exercises.

You can schedule for a specific time each day or for different times of the day. Doing yoga in the morning gives children the energy to start the day, yoga during the day refreshes them so they can carry on, and yoga at the end of the day helps them to release tension.

One of the teacher's most important roles is to choose exercises that suit the development level of the children. Be flexible if it becomes clear that they are not enjoying an activity you planned or are unable to do it.

Make sure that you are thoroughly familiar with the exercises and have tried them yourself before the lesson. It is a good idea to do the entire lesson—including any stories, songs, or rhymes—at least once yourself so that you know how it all fits together. Then you can decide which activities are best for the children you're working with and make any appropriate adjustments before class.

There are different ways of teaching a game, and which one you choose depends on your preference, the type of exercise, and the group you are working with. In some cases, you can simply do the lesson with the children, encouraging them to join in with your example and with minimal verbal instruction. If an exercise needs more explanation, however, it is better to carefully explain the exercise and demonstrate it first. That way, when the children know what to do ahead of time, they are more likely to join in, do it properly, and enjoy themselves.

When working with children you need to be aware of so many things at the same time. Are they all joining in? Do they know in which order to do things? Are they doing it correctly? Do they need more instruction or demonstration? Are they enjoying themselves? Are any of the exercises too difficult?

You can build up a lesson bit by bit, introducing the more simple games first and gradually introducing the more complex exercises.

Tips

Scattered throughout the book are a number of practical tips. Some are more general while others are specific to the lesson. These tips should not be seen as hard and fast directions; they are mainly suggestions intended as support. Most come from years of practicing yoga and working with kids, as will be evident when you come across them in the book.

Rules

Children prefer to know in advance what they will be doing. Giving them clear direction on how to behave during the lesson will help them to feel more secure, will encourage them to participate, and will make the lesson go smoothly. These rules should be simple, as few as possible, and appropriate to the ages of the children you are teaching. It is also important to be consistent and to use a gentle and friendly manner when explaining and enforcing the rules.

If you are teaching a class of children other than your own, you might want to put the rules on paper and give them to the parents to go over with their children before class. Do not assume, however, that the parents will apply the same rules at home. If you are working with children who can read, you can also make a poster of the rules and display it in the exercise area.

One rule that is essential to any yoga class for children is this one: "Be quiet." It is also important to make sure the children understand that you are giving the lesson and you decide which exercises are going to be done in which order and when the kids should change partners. These two rules will ensure that the children listen well and quietly follow your instructions. Of course, you may want to make other rules too—such as to be respectful of one another and not to eat or chew gum during class. Just remember to keep the rules simple and the lesson playful.

From time to time you may need to bend the rules a little, but you must ensure that it is quiet when it should be, for instance, when reading a story. You can also agree in advance to allow those children who do not want to join in to sit quietly somewhere and perhaps draw or read a book while the other children participate in the activity. This should not be presented as a punishment, but rather as a practical solution to a child's needs.

Tuning In to the Group

Try to adapt the tone of your lesson to the personalities and moods of the children. A good way of doing this is to start the lesson with a group discussion. This gives the children your attention and encourages them to talk about things they want to say. I can sometimes determine that a particular exercise won't fit because, at that time with those children, a more gentle or a more robust exercise is needed.

The children's difficulty in being quiet and in paying attention are common challenges for yoga teachers, and the two go hand in hand. Children are easily distracted, and too much noise impedes their ability to concentrate. Quietness begins with yourself, so make sure that you are quiet and relaxed when teaching a yoga class to children. If you are annoyed or irritated, children will certainly pick up on it, even if you try to hide it. When you are quiet within, they will notice that too. Set a good example, and they will follow.

The Teacher's Attitude

As a teacher, your attitude as you stand in front of the class is key to the success of the lesson. If you put too much effort into achieving a certain goal or too much time into an exercise to improve their skills or too much emphasis on their performance, that intensity can quickly diminish the children's natural enthusiasm. The art is to find the right balance between playfulness and seriousness, which begins by developing a positive attitude toward the children's behavior.

Asking yourself the following questions will help you assess the effectiveness of your attitude:

1. Are the children learning and developing at a satisfactory pace?

2. Am I overstimulating or understimulating them?

3. Are my expectations realistic?

4. What do I mean if I say something is good or well done?

5. Can I be flexible with the children's own contributions without losing control of the lesson?

6. Do I know the children well enough to give them the correct level of exercises?

Observation and Reflection

Carefully observing the children during the lesson and reflecting on what you see is a good way to assess how well your approach is working. It is also a great source of information for the next lessons, in relation both to your approach and to the program itself. By watching the children you can see all kinds of discrepancies that you can address immediately, sometimes during a certain exercise, or later, at the end of class or in another lesson. This observation and reflection process gives you a better picture of what the children can and can't do at this phase in their development, how well they follow direction, and their social behavior.

Here are several things you can observe and ask yourself during the class to evaluate how the children are using the exercises:

1. Are they engaged by and connecting with the theme?

2. Are they using their own ideas?

3. Are they concentrating and absorbed in the lesson?

4. Can they get into the swing of it and enjoy it sufficiently?

5. To what extent are they cooperating?

6. Are they able to react to each other and in what way?

Key to the Icons Used in the Exercises and Games

To help you find games suitable for a particular situation, each game is coded with symbols, or icons, that tell you the following things about the activity at a glance:

- the size of the group needed
- if props are required
- if children will exercise on a mat
- if a large space is required
- if musical accompaniment is required
- if physical contact is or might be involved

These are explained in more detail below.

The size of the group needed. While some games require partners, you can play many of the games with any sized group.

 = The whole group plays together

 = The children play individually, so any size group can play

 = The children play in pairs

If props are required. Many of the games require no special props. In some cases, though, items such as balloons, crystals, or other objects are integral to running and playing a game. Games requiring props are flagged with the following icon, and the necessary materials are listed under the Props heading.

 = Props needed

If an exercise mat is required. Children exercise and do yoga postures on the floor in some of the games. In those games, a mat, rug, towel, or blanket might be used for the children's comfort and safety.

 = Players will exercise on mats

If a large space is required. Almost all yoga games may be played in a relatively small space. However, a large space is ideal for some of the games. The few games that require a large amount of space are marked with the following icon:

 = Large space needed

If music is required. Only a few games in this book require the playing of recorded music. Several games include suggestions for suitable music. For instance, we might recommend music with Eastern themes or African drums.

 = Music required

If physical contact is or might be involved. Although a certain amount of body contact might be acceptable in certain environments, the following icon has been inserted at the top of any exercise that might involve anything from a small amount of contact to minor collisions. You can figure out in advance if the game is suitable for your participants and/or environment.

 = Physical contact likely

The Games

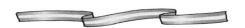

Rise and Shine

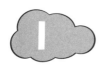 # Feeling the Sun

Tell the children: *The sun has risen, and the sunbeams shine through the window onto your face.*

- *Lie on your back with your arms by your sides.*
- *Feel the warmth of the sunbeams on your body.*
- *Feel the sun warming your face, your chest, your tummy, your arms, your hands, your legs, and your feet.*

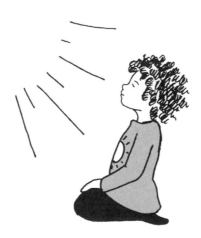

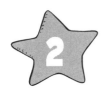

Giant Yawn

any size

Tell the children to make a giant yawn. To do this, tell them to:

- *Stand up straight.*
- *Raise your arms over your head and stretch yourself out.*
- *Open your mouth wide, and say "aaaaaaaahh."*

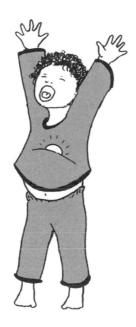

❖ ❖ ❖ ❖ ❖ ❖ **Your body feels deliciously warm.**
Next, you will wake up your body,
starting with your fingers. ❖ ❖ ❖ ❖ ❖ ❖

Waking Fingers

any size

Instruct the children as follows:

- *Sit up straight.*

- *Hold your hand in front of you with your palm turned toward your face.*

- *Make a fist. All your fingers are closed—they are still sleeping.*

- *Wake up your fingers by making them stand up one by one. Start with your thumb, then your index finger, your middle finger, your ring finger, and the little finger.*

- *If one of your fingers doesn't want to wake up, help it with your other hand.*

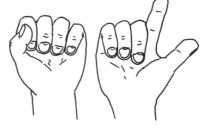

- *Now, wake up the fingers on your other hand.*

Tip: While playing the game, the children can sing this song—saying the appropriate name (Thumbkin, Pointer, Middleman, Ringman, Pinkie), raising the appropriate finger at "Here I am," and hiding the hand behind the back at "Run away":

Where is Thumbkin, where is Thumbkin?

Here I am, here I am.

How are you this morning?

Very well, I thank you.

Run away, run away.

❖ ❖ ❖ ❖ ❖ ❖ **Now let's wake up your entire body.** ❖ ❖ ❖ ❖ ❖ ❖

Shaking Loose

Tell the children to do the following:

- *Get out of bed and stand up straight.*
- *Shake your hands loose from the wrist—one at a time.*
- *Shake one arm and then the other.*
- *Shake one foot and then the other.*
- *Shake one leg and then the other.*
- *Shake your whole body loose.*

 # Good Morning

Say to the children:

- *Look around you to see who else is awake.*
- *Smile at everyone and say "good morning."*

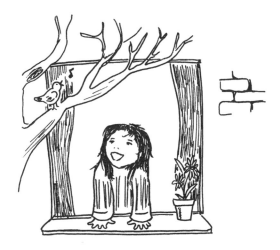

Freshen Up

Now it's time to get ready for our big
adventure. Let's start by brushing our teeth.

Brushing Teeth

any size

Ask the children to act out brushing their teeth as follows:

- *Move your toothbrush (your index finger) back and forth in front of your mouth.*
- *Pretend to take a mouthful of water and fill up your cheeks with it.*
- *Spit the water into the sink.*
- *Show your nice clean teeth to your friends and give a broad grin.*

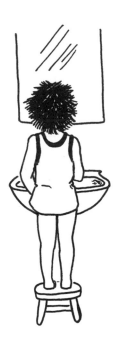

Now it's time for a refreshing shower.

 **7**

Showering

Instruct the children as follows:

- *With your fingers, imitate the drops of water falling on your body.*
- *Start by tapping your fingers on your head and work your way down over your neck, shoulders, arms, chest, tummy, bottom, and legs.*
- *You can also hear the drops of water; listen carefully while you are tapping your fingers.*

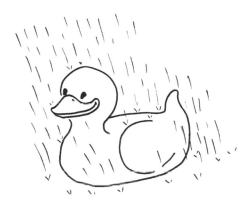

❀ ❀ ❀ ❀ ❀ ❀ **You are all wet**
from your shower,
so start drying yourself off. ❀ ❀ ❀ ❀ ❀ ❀

Drying Off

any size

Props: A piece of paper towel for each child

Say:

- *Sit up tall with your legs spread apart.*
- *Place the paper towel on the floor between your legs.*
- *Use the toes on one foot to pick up the paper towel.*
- *With your hand, grab the paper towel from your toes.*
- *Dry one leg from bottom to top and then the other.*
- *What other parts of your body need drying? Dry those too.*

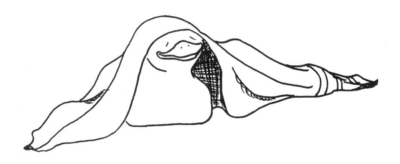

❖ ❖ ❖ ❖ ❖ ❖ **It's time to get dressed.** ❖ ❖ ❖ ❖ ❖ ❖

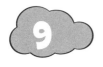 # Getting Dressed

Divide the group into pairs. Tell the children:

- *Decide who will be the "mirror" and who will get dressed.*
- *Stand facing your partner.*
- *If you are the child getting dressed, look in your "mirror" and pretend you are dressing.*
- *If you are the mirror, copy your partner's movements.*
- *Change places and repeat.*

Tip: The children can try the following movements:

- combing hair
- putting on pants and shirts
- putting on socks and shoes
- putting on jackets and caps
- putting on scarves and mittens

Now you are fresh, clean, and ready to start the day.

To the Zoo

It's a lovely day today.
You are going to the zoo.

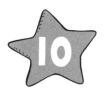

10 Let's Talk about It

Prepare the children for the visit to the zoo by asking the following questions:

- *Who has been to the zoo?*
- *Which animals did you see or smell or touch?*
- *Which is your favorite animal?*
- *Would you like to be an animal? Which one?*

Before you leave,
make sure you have packed
everything you'll need
for your zoo adventure.

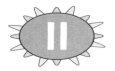 # I'm Going to the Zoo and I'm Taking

Say: *Let's make a list of what you want to take to the zoo.*

- *Sit in a semicircle.*
- *I'll begin: "I'm going to the zoo, and I'm taking sandwiches."*
- *Now, go down the row and each of you, one by one, repeat the sentence and add something you want to bring to the zoo. For example, "I'm going to the zoo, and I'm taking sandwiches and **a drink**."*
- *When it's your turn, repeat all the items the other children want to bring and then add yours.*

Tip: If you are playing with only a few children, you can do two or three rounds of this game.

**You are so happy
to be going to the zoo
that you dance for joy.**

Zoo Day Dance

any size

Along with the children, sing the following song and make the movements that go with it:

1. *Make a circle big and round (bring your arms up from your sides).*

2. *Bend right over to the ground.*

3. *Lie on your tummy like a snake (cobra posture).*

4. *Stretch your arms out very long (arms above your head).*

5. *Rest a moment, very quiet (arms under your head).*

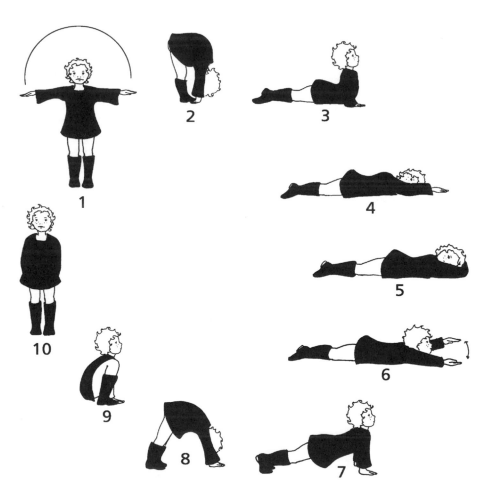

6. Change into a crocodile (crocodile posture).

7. Push yourself up from the ground (plank posture).

8. Sit up like a dog (dog posture).

9. Jump forward like a rabbit (frog posture).

10. We're going off to the zoo! (stand up). That's great!

❖ ❖ ❖ ❖ ❖ ❖ **Let's walk to the bus station,**
where a bus is waiting
to take us to the zoo. ❖ ❖ ❖ ❖ ❖ ❖

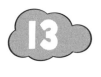 # Walking to the Bus

Say to the children:

- *Stand up straight.*
- *Walk in place.*
- *Now walk faster.*
- *Slow down and then come to a stop.*

❖ ❖ ❖ ❖ ❖ ❖ **Now we can**
board the bus
and go to the zoo! ❖ ❖ ❖ ❖ ❖ ❖

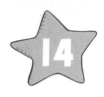 **14** # Riding the Bus

Tell the children:

- *Sit on the floor in a row, one passenger behind another, with your legs stretched out in front of you.*

- *Bring your hands in front of you and point your elbows outward.*

- *Make circles with each of your arms in a forward direction, like the wheels on the bus, going round and round.*

- *At the same time, scoot your bottom back and forth a little. The bus is now moving forward.*

- *While you ride along in the bus, sing this song:*

> *The wheels on the bus go round and round,*
> *Round and round, round and round.*
> *The wheels on the bus go round and round,*
> *All through the town.*

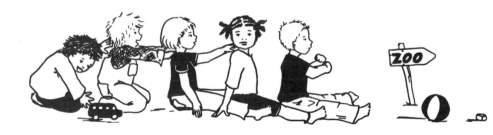

Entering the Zoo

○○ ○○ ○○ **Hurrah! We've arrived at the zoo.**
Before we can go in, we must get our tickets. ○○ ○○ ○○ ○○

 **15** # Through the Gate

whole
group

Teach the children how to play the game as follows:

- One pair of children stands face-to face.
- Those two children clasp hands and raise their arms above their heads to form a "bridge."
- The other children stand in line behind the "bridge."

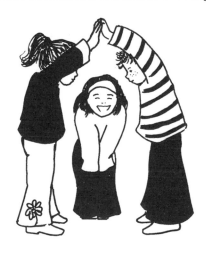

- The children standing in line walk through the gate one at a time.
- The last two children to walk through the gate replace the two "gatekeepers." They stand facing one another and form a bridge with their hands.
- The first pair of gatekeepers walk through the gate, one by one.

The game can continue until everyone has had a chance to be a gatekeeper.

❖ ❖ ❖ ❖ ❖ ❖ Our zoo adventure begins on a footbridge. From here, you can watch the animals do what animals do. ❖ ❖ ❖ ❖ ❖ ❖

16 Crossing the Footbridge

Tell the children:
- *Stand at the edge of your mat. This is the footbridge.*
- *Carefully walk one foot after the other (like on a balance beam) to the middle of the footbridge.*
- *Stand with your feet side by side and look all around you. What animals do you see?*
- *Let's go see the animals now. Walk to the end of the bridge and make a big jump. Now you are in the zoo!*

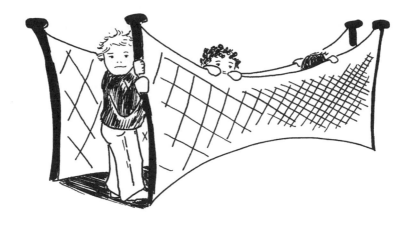

Tip: Instead of walking across the mat one foot in front of the other, the children can walk on their toes, their heels, or the insides or outsides of their feet. You can also ask them which other ways they know to get across—jumping, hopping, shuffling, or stamping.

A walk through the zoo is like a journey around the world. Along the way you will discover all kinds of strong, fascinating, and agile animals from many different countries. In the wild, you could never get as close to these creatures as you can at the zoo.

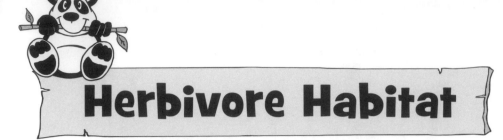

Herbivore Habitat

First, you come to a place that looks like the savannah. Here, you will find <u>herbivores</u>— plant-eating animals, such as giraffes and zebras. The first animals you see are giraffes.

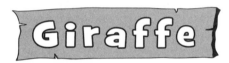

Giraffe

Giraffes are so tall they can eat leaves from the treetops. When giraffes walk, they swing their necks back and forth.

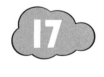 # Looking for Leaves

Say: *Let's look for leaves in the tall trees.*
- *Stand up straight and stretch your arms above your head.*
- *Make yourself as tall as a giraffe.*

- *Stick your thumbs up and rest them against your head so that they look like horns.*
- *Walk around with a straight back and with your arms and legs stretched out.*
- *As you walk, look left and right, moving your head back and forth.*
- *Search for juicy leaves high up in the trees.*
- *Stick out your tongue to pick the leaves.*
- *As you walk around, sing this song [to the tune of "They Fly through the Air with the Greatest of Ease"]:*

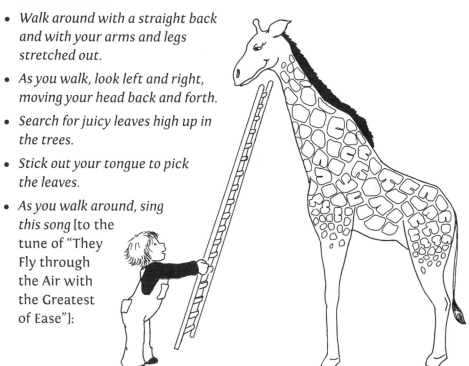

The yellow giraffe is as tall as can be,
He munches on leaves at the tops of the trees,
His neck is quite long and his legs are long too,
He can run faster than his friends at the zoo.

A long neck is very useful for picking leaves from the high branches, but it makes eating grass or drinking water from a pool very difficult. The giraffe has to spread his front legs far apart for his head to reach the ground.

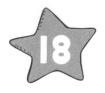 # Drinking Water

Ask the children: *Can you drink water like a giraffe?*
- *Stand up with your legs wide apart.*
- *Bend over and try to get your head as close to the ground as you can.*
- *Put your hands on the ground far apart.*
- *Imagine that you are drinking water just like a giraffe.*
- *Stay bent over for a minute and then slowly stand up again.*
- *Repeat once or twice.*

Giraffes have very long tongues that are very flexible and very sensitive. That is useful when you have to pick up small things with it!

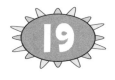 # Tongue Stretch

Instruct the children as follows:
- *Stick out your tongue are far as it will go.*
- *Try to touch the tip of your nose with your tongue.*
- *Now roll it up into your mouth.*
- *Can you curl your tongue too?*

Giraffes run very fast, but they have an unusual way of doing it. Both the front and back legs on the left side move forward at the same time; then the front and back legs on the right side move together at the same time. With each step, the giraffe pushes off with one or the other front leg. Try to walk and then run like a giraffe.

Galloping

 any size

Say to the children:

- *Stand with your legs apart.*
- *Lean forward and place your hands flat on the floor in front of you.*
- *Lift and move your left hand and your left leg forward at the same time.*
- *Lift and move your right hand your right leg forward at the same time.*
- *Take several steps forward, again moving your left hand and leg at the same time and then your right hand and leg at the same time. Try to go a little faster with each step.*

A giraffe's back is as steep as a sliding board, because its front legs are so much longer than its back legs.

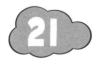 # Look, I'm a Slide!

Ask the children to make their bodies into slides by reading them the instructions below aloud:

- *Sit up straight with your legs stretched out in front of you.*
- *Place your hands on the floor behind you with your fingers pointing backward.*
- *Raise your buttocks off the ground and stand on your hands and heels.*
- *Hold this position for as long as you can.*
- *Slowly sit back down.*

The path you are walking on leads to a watering place. There you can watch the zebras from very close by.

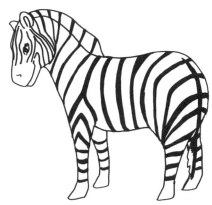
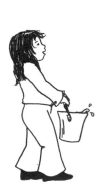

❖ ❖ ❖ ❖ ❖ ❖ **Zebras can turn their ears up, down, backward, and forward so they can hear the smallest sounds. This is very important in the wild, where they need to hear their enemies.** ❖ ❖ ❖ ❖ ❖ ❖

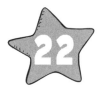 **22** # Twitching Ears

Say: *Can you move your ears in all directions? Some people can wiggle their ears, but most of us need a little help to move our ears.*

- *Sit up straight.*
- *Take your ear between your thumb and index finger.*
- *Gently move your ear to the side, up, down, forward, and backward.*

❀ ❀ ❀ ❀ ❀ ❀ **Zebras walk and run
like horses, and they kick
like donkeys. Let's see
if you can, too!** ❀ ❀ ❀ ❀ ❀ ❀

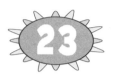 # High-Stepping

Guide the children as follows:

- *Get down on your hands and knees.*
- *Lift your right hand and your left leg and move them one step forward at the same time.*
- *Lift your left hand and your right leg and move them one step forward at the same time.*
- *Repeat this a few times, trying to move a little faster with each step.*

 # Kicking

Ask the children to kick like a zebra would:

- *Stand on your hands and feet with your knees bent.*
- *Lean forward a little to put most of your weight on your hands.*
- *Kick your right foot up and back, followed immediately by your left leg.*
- *When both feet come down, kick your left foot up and back, followed immediately by your right foot.*
- *Repeat a few times.*

- *Can you make a sound like a zebra while you're kicking? Zebras bray like donkeys and snort like horses.*

Tip: Make sure to space the children far apart so they don't accidentally kick one another.

Your adventure at the zoo continues. Next you come to the elephant enclosure.

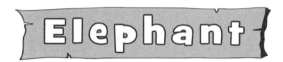

The elephants have just been brought in by their keeper. Did you know that an elephant can eat a whole wheelbarrow full of food at one meal? With a friend, you can pretend to be a zoo keeper and bring food to the elephants in a wheelbarrow.

25 Wheelbarrow Walk

Divide the children into two groups: "wheelbarrows" and "zoo keepers," and have each wheelbarrow partner up with a zoo keeper. Teach the children how to play the game as follows:

- *If you are a wheelbarrow, lie on your tummy with your hands flat on the floor.*
- *If you are a zoo keeper, pick up your partner's feet.*
- *Wheelbarrow, as the "zoo keeper" lifts your feet, stretch out your arms and lift your body up from the floor.*
- *Take a few steps forward—with "wheelbarrows" walking on your hands and "zoo keepers" following behind still holding onto your partner's legs.*
- *Switch roles with your partner and play the game again.*

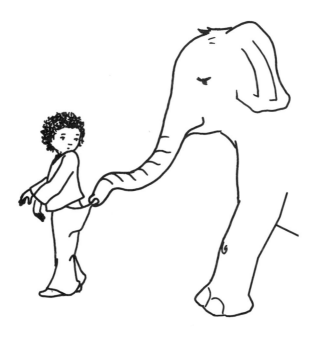

Some elephants are so hungry that they go off by themselves without the herd to look for food. Elephants use the pointy ends of their trunks like fingers to pick up all kinds of things—apples, bananas, melons, even small things like peanuts.

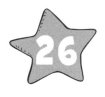 # Searching for Food

Props: A small ball for each child

Say:

- *Stand up straight.*
- *Hold your nose with one hand.*
- *Put your other hand through the opening in the crook of your arm.*
- *Bend over and try to pick up an apple (ball) from the ground.*
- *See if you can bring the apple (ball) to your mouth.*

Tip: Place a few small balls on the floor around the room to represent apples.

Elephants scratch themselves with their trunks. It is very easy for them to scratch their heads and even their backs; they don't need to ask anyone for help.

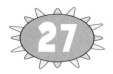 # Back Scratch

Tell the children to try scratching their own backs:

- *Make a trunk like you did in the previous exercise.*
- *Now reach your "trunk" (arm) around and see if you can scratch your back.*
- *Change your trunk to the other arm and scratch the other side of your back.*

Elephants use their trunks
to touch their friends.
That's how they say
hello to each other.

Hello, Friend!

whole
group

Have the children pretend to be elephants that are greeting their friends:

- *Stand in a circle and look around you.*
- *Look each other in the eye and say, "Hello, it's good to see you."*
- *Make a trunk like you did before.*
- *Gently "shake trunks" (hands) with your neighbors.*

Elephants have sloping soles
with a thick springy pad under their
feet. They actually walk on their tip-toes,
so quietly that you can barely hear their
footsteps. When they walk together,
they often hold hands —
or rather, each other's
trunks and tails.

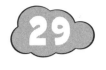 **29** **Hiking** with the **Herd**

 whole group

Say to the children: *Let's all go for a stroll!*

- *Stand in a line, one behind the other.*
- *Bend over and reach your right arm backward through your legs.*
- *Catch the left hand of the person behind you. You are now holding onto their "trunk," and their trunk is holding onto your "tail." In the process, your "trunk" holds onto the "tail" of the person in front of you.*
- *Walk on your toes, one person behind the other, very quietly.*
- *While you are walking, sing this song:*

> *Elephants walk along the trails*
> *With trunks holding onto tails,*
> *When they walk it never fails*
> *They hold hands by holding tails.*

Tip: You can make up a simple tune for this song or borrow a tune from a popular children's song, such as "Here We Go 'Round the Mulberry Bush."

As we continue our journey through the zoo, we come to the rhinoceroses. Together with the elephants, rhinos are some of the biggest mammals in the world.

Rhinoceros

Rhinos can turn their ears in all directions, so they can even hear sounds behind them clearly. They also have a very good sense of smell. Let's see if you can tell where the sounds are coming from.

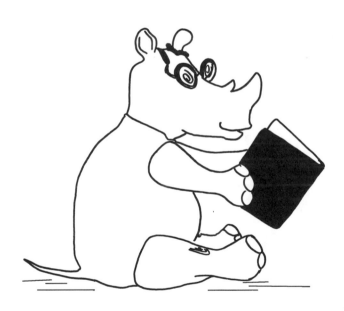

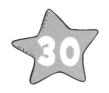 **Hearing**

Teach the children how to play the game as follows:

- All but one of the children sit in a circle. One child—the "noise-maker"—remains standing.
- The seated children close their eyes and cup their hands over their ears while the noisemaker finds a hiding place.
- The noisemaker makes a soft sound—such as snoring, puffing, or grunting.
- The other children point to where the sound is coming from.
- Repeat several times, allowing different children to be the noise-maker.

 **Smelling**

 any size

Props: A few aromatic items with varying scents, such as flowers, soap, pine needles, vanilla, peanut butter, and lemon

Ask the children to discover how they breathe when they smell different scents:

- *Sit up straight.*
- *Smell each of the items, one by one. Take a few breaths of fresh air between each scent you inhale.*
- *What do you notice about your breath when you smell each scent? Do you breathe differently with smells you like than smells you don't like?*

Rhinos are often visited by tick birds. These birds use their claws to pick the ticks, flies, and dead skin from the rhino's hide, which they then eat. Rhinos are happy to get a clean-up by these hungry birds!

 # 32 **Feeling**

pairs

Divide the group into pairs. Say: *Can you feel the bird on your back?*

- *Decide who will be the "rhino" and who will be the "bird."*
- *Sit one behind the other, with the bird in back and the rhino in front.*
- *If you are the bird, use your thumb and forefinger to pick "bugs" off your partner's back.*
- *If you are the rhino, feel the gentle touch of your partner's fingers.*
- *Change places and play the game again.*

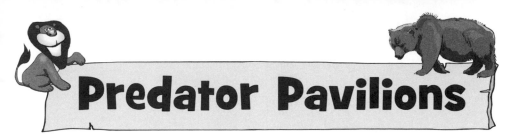

Predator Pavilions

As we continue our zoo adventure, we reach the place where the great hunters live. You can watch these predators from the safety of the observation decks.

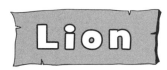

Lion

First you come across a pride of lions. Male lions have a large thick mane, sharp teeth and claws, and very strong muscles. When they open their mouths, they can make a deafening roar. No wonder they call the lion the king of the jungle.

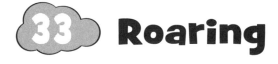

33 Roaring

any size

Instruct the children as follows: *Feel that you are as strong and powerful as a lion, and make sure everyone hears you roar.*

- *Sit on your haunches with your bottom on your heels.*
- *Put your hands flat on the ground and stretch your arms.*
- *Open your eyes wide, stick out your tongue, and roar: Rrraarrhh!*

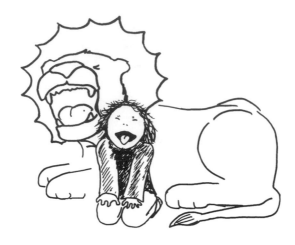

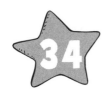 **Young lions often play tag in the savannah. Would you like to play tag with your friends?**

34 Catch Me If You Can!

Teach the children how to play the game as follows:

- Decide who will be "It" (the "tagger") and who will be the "rescuer."
- The rest of the children spread out and move all around the room.
- The tagger tries to "catch" as many "cubs" as they can by gently tapping them.
- When a cub is "caught," that child sits down wherever they are tagged.
- The rescuer can "release" the captured cubs by tapping them gently on the shoulder.

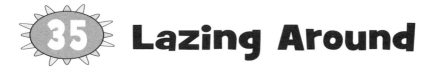 **Lions love to lie around doing nothing, stretched out in the strangest positions just enjoying the sun.**

 # Lazing Around

Ask the children to show how many ways they can lie down.

Lions can show each other what they mean with their body, scent, or touch.

Body Talk

Divide the group into pairs. Tell the children: *Show another person what you mean without talking.*

- *Stand facing your partner.*
- *Take turns using a body movement to silently "say" something to the other person.*
- *Say aloud what your partner has "said" with his or her body talk.*

Tip: Give the children a few examples of body talk, such as: "good" (thumbs up), "come here" (beckon with forefinger), "be quiet" (forefinger to lips), "I don't know" (shrug shoulders), and "surprise" (raised eyebrows).

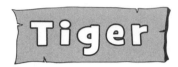 **A little farther on in the Predator Pavilions you find the tigers.**

Tiger

Tigers belong to the cat family, which you can tell by their sharp teeth and claws. They also have thick cushions on the soles of their feet that allow them to walk very quietly so antelope and other animals do not hear them coming.

37 Slinking

Say to the children:

- *Get down on your hands and knees.*
- *Slink around like a tiger.*
- *Spread your fingers and show your claws!*

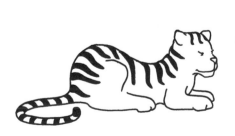 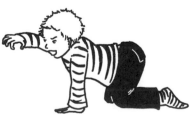

Tigers live alone—except for mamas and their young cubs. They urinate to mark the edges of their territory to let others know that a tiger already lives there.

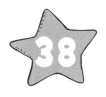

Marking Territory

any size

Read the following instructions to the children:

- *Get down on your hands and knees.*
- *Lift one of your legs up to the side, like a dog lifts its leg to urinate on a bush.*
- *Pretend you are urinating to mark your space, just like a tiger.*

Tigers hide their cubs—usually in tall grass or thick vegetation— to protect them from other predators. Their striped coats provide a camouflage, helping the cubs to blend into their surroundings.

 # Hide and Peek

Say: *Pretend you are a tiger cub hiding in the thick brush. Use your hands, books, or desks as things to hide behind, or move your body to camouflage, or hide, yourself.*

- *Hide your tummy.*
- *On the signal, let your tummy be seen again.*
- *Hide your feet.*
- *On the signal, let your feet be seen again.*
- *Hide your lips.*
- *On the signal, let your lips be seen again.*

Tip: You can instruct the children to hide and reveal any and as many parts of the body as you wish.

❖ ❖ ❖ ❖ ❖ ❖ **Now you've arrived at the bear pit. To keep the bears strong and healthy, their keepers make them work for their food. Every morning, the keepers hide apples and bread in tree trunks and among the rocks. Sometimes they even smear peanut butter and syrup on the rocks.** ❖ ❖ ❖ ❖ ❖ ❖

Bear

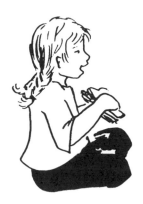 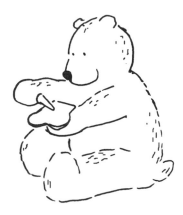

✿ ✿ ✿ ✿ ✿ ✿ **Just like humans, bears put down
their whole foot when they walk,
placing their heel on the ground first
and then rocking forward on the soles of
their feet. Of course, bears have four feet,
instead of two. To walk, they first put
the two paws on one side of their bodies
forward, with the hind paw moving first
and the front paw lifting just before the
hind paw lands, and then they do the same
with the two paws on the other side of their
bodies (e.g., they start with the left hind
paw, then the left front, the right hind, the
right front, and then the left hind again).** ✿ ✿ ✿ ✿ ✿ ✿

40 Walking in the Woods

Guide the children as follows: *Walk through the forest looking for food. Bears will eat almost anything, but they especially love honey, fish, berries, and fruit.*

- *Get down on your hands and knees.*
- *Walk forward moving your left leg first, then your left arm, your right leg, your right arm, and your left leg again.*
- *Go around the room searching for food.*
- *When you find something yummy to eat, stop for a picnic.*
- *Use your front "paws" to grab and eat your food.*

Tip: Encourage the kids to use different body movements—for example, to lean over a river for fish, to crawl in a log for honey, and to stand on hind legs to pluck fruit from a bush or tree.

Bears are very strong and have long, sharp teeth and claws. Although they usually stay away from people, they can be very dangerous, so don't tease them at the zoo and never go near any bear, including cubs, in the wild.

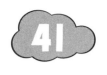 # Beware of the Bear

Teach the children how to play the game as follows:

- Divide the children into two groups: those who will play "bears" and those who will play "hunters."
- The children act out the movements as they listen to the story (below).

*A **hunter** goes out to the woods on a bear hunt (walk in place).*

*He hears a **bear** roaring (roar).*

*The **hunter** drops his gun in fright (stamp feet on floor).*

*The **bear** comes closer and closer (crawl toward hunters).*

*The **hunter** drops to the ground (lie down on back).*

*The **hunter** pretends to be dead (lie very still).*

*The **bear** comes right up to the hunter (crawl to a hunter).*

*The **bear** investigates the hunter by prodding him gently and looking to see whether he is alive (snuffle around the hunter).*

*The **hunters** must not laugh (be very quiet).*

*Fooled by the clever hunter, the **bear** walks away (crawl away).*

Our next stop is the enclosure where a skulk of foxes live in separate dens. Foxes usually live and hunt alone, except for a mama with babies.

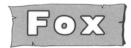
Fox

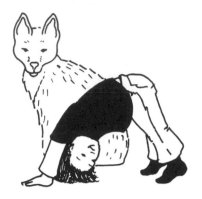

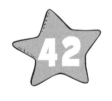 **Foxes know a good trick to catch rabbits. They start jumping around and dancing in circles. The mesmerized rabbits don't notice that the fox is coming closer and closer. Try enchanting your friends with a dance.**

42 Dance of Enchantment

whole group

Music: Dance

Teach the children how to play the game as follows:

- Divide the children into two groups: (1) those who will play "foxes" and (2) those who will play "rabbits."
- The foxes try to entrance the rabbits with their dance.
- The rabbits squat on their haunches (sitting on feet), watching and staying very still.

- When the music stops, the foxes tag the rabbits.
- Then the children can change places and repeat the game.

Foxes usually sleep above ground in a hidden spot, such as in a hollow log, a rock pile, or in a burrow dug into the ground. This is called a lair or a den. When foxes wake up, they stretch just like dogs.

 # **Morning Fox Trot**

Ask the children to listen to the story below and act out the movements:

The fox lies curled up, fast asleep (lie on side with chin and knees to chest, eyes closed).

He opens his eyes, lifts his head, and looks around.

He stretches his back leg and then his front leg.

He stands up on all fours (on hands and knees).

He swings his tail back and forth (wiggle bottom).

The fox is now awake and ready to go hunting.

He walks about (crawl on hands and knees).

He sees a rabbit hole and looks down (on hands and feet, bottom in air, head upside down and looking at navel).

He takes a closer look (sit with bottom on heels and bend forward from waist until chest and belly rest on legs).

The fox continues his walk (on hands and knees) and greets the other foxes in his own fashion (nods, sniffs, yips, nuzzles, etc.)

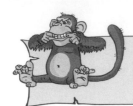

Ape Cages

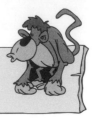

You have arrived
at the ape exhibit,
where first you see the chimps.

Chimpanzee

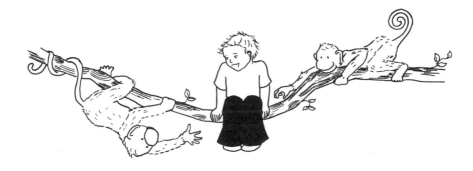

Young chimps love playing with
their friends, hanging in trees,
and rolling around on the ground.
They also enjoy jumping and fighting.
They scream loud about the smallest things,
and they constantly show off what
they can do and how brave they are.

Jumping

Tell the children: *Jump like a chimp and show how brave you are.*

- *Form your hands into loose fists.*
- *Bend over forward with your arms and legs straight and place the flat part of your fingers (knuckles) on the ground.*
- *Hop up and down so that your hands and feet leave the floor at the same time. Make sure to bend your knees each time you come down.*
- *Do the chimp-jump again eight times in a row.*

Tip: Encourage the children to make chimp noises and faces.

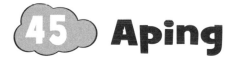 **Chimps learn a lot from each other by watching and copying what other chimps do.**

Aping

pairs

Divide the group into pairs and say to the children: *See what you can learn by copying a friend.*

- *Decide who will be the "little chimp" and who will be the "big chimp."*
- *Stand facing your partner.*
- *If you are the big chimp, do something chimp-like, such as scratching your armpits, shaking your arms, chattering your teeth, pursing your lips, or bouncing up and down.*
- *If you are the little chimp, copy your partner's movement.*
- *Big chimp, repeat your first movement and add another one.*

- *Little chimp, copy your partner's first and second movements.*
- *Big chimp, repeat your first and second movements and add another movement.*
- *Little chimp, copy all three movements.*

Tip: After two or three movements, the children can change places, so everyone gets the chance to ape (i.e., copy) movements. As another option, the children can ape the teacher instead of each other. How many movements can the children remember?

A baby chimp is born with a red, wrinkly face that looks a lot like an old man.

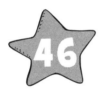 # 46 **Funny Face**

Read the following instructions aloud:
- *Make a scrunched-up, wrinkly face like a baby chimp.*
- *Look at your friends and give them each a great, big, goofy, wrinkly-faced grin.*

Mama chimps love to take their babies everywhere with them. The baby hangs on tightly to the mama's neck or back. Sometimes the baby even hangs under the mama's tummy.

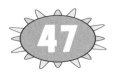 **47** **Out with Mama**

Props: A baby doll or stuffed animal for each child

Instruct the children as follows:

- *Pick up your baby and hold it with one arm.*
- *Make a loose fist with your other hand.*
- *Stand with knees slightly bent, bend over, and rest the flat part of your fingers (knuckles) on the floor.*
- *Walk around the room like a chimp, holding the baby close to your chest.*

Chimps love to pick fleas off each other. This is a way of grooming, playing with, or comforting one another—like when humans brush one another's hair or get a facial.

 48 **Grooming**

Divide the group into pairs and have the children pretend to pick fleas off another chimp.

- *Decide who will be the "groomer" and who will be the "friend."*
- *Sit with the groomer in back and the friend in front.*
- *If you are the groomer, use your forefinger and thumb, gently "pick fleas" from your partner's hair.*

- *If you're the friend, feel the gentle, caring touch of your partner's fingers.*
- *Change places and play the game again.*

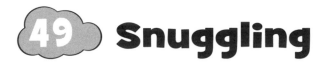 **Small chimps sleep on their mother's chest. Snuggled against the mama chimp's soft, warm fur, the baby quickly falls fast asleep.**

49 Snuggling

pairs

Divide the group into pairs and guide the children through this activity as follows:

- *Decide who will be the "mama chimp" and who will be the "baby chimp."*
- *Sit one behind the other, with the mama in back and the baby in front.*
- *If you're the mama, stretch your legs around your partner.*
- *If you're the baby, gently lean back against your partner's chest.*
- *Babies, feel the warmth, breathing, and heartbeat of your partner.*
- *Mamas, feel the warmth and breathing of your partner.*
- *Change places and play the game again.*

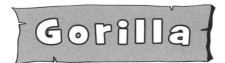

Gorilla

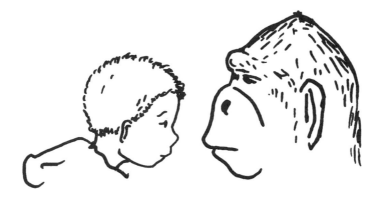

❖ ❖ ❖ ❖ ❖ ❖ **Gorillas use their faces to show how they are feeling. If they put their tongue on their nose, they are feeling uneasy. If their mouth is open, like a smile, they are happy, but gorillas who show their teeth are running out of patience.** ❖ ❖ ❖ ❖ ❖

50 How Am I Feeling?

any size

Say: *How are you feeling today? Show everyone how you feel.*

- *Make your face look happy.*
- *Look sad.*
- *Look angry.*
- *Look shy.*

**If a strange gorilla turns up, the leader of the group
will act big and tough to show how strong he is
and to let the stranger know he had better leave.**

 # Chest Beating

Ask the children to show how strong they are by having them beat their chests with their fists and say "oo-oo, oo-oo, oo-oo, oo-oo."

**Gorillas walk on two feet by balancing
on the knuckles of their hands.**

 # Knuckle Walking

Say: *Can you walk like a gorilla?*
- *Stand with your feet a little bit apart and your knees slightly bent.*
- *Curl your hands into loose fists.*
- *Put your arms out in front of you, bend forward, and place the flat part of the backs of your fingers (knuckles) on the floor.*
- *Move forward by pushing off with your right hand as you take a step with your left foot.*
- *Take another step forward, this time pushing off with your left hand and moving your right foot.*
- *Knuckle-walk a few more steps.*

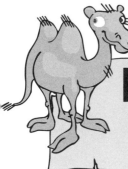

Desert Animal Compound

In the desert, it rarely rains and water is hard to find. The desert can be very hot during the day and very cold at night. So it is not easy to survive there. Yet some animals can live in the desert without drinking a drop of water!

Camel

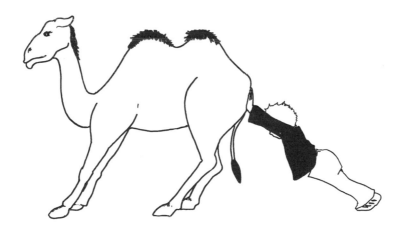

The first animal you come across in the desert area is the camel. Camels walk along with a swinging gait.

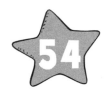 **Hip Walk**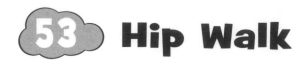

Tell the children: *Try walking like a camel, with your hips rocking gently from side to side.*

- *Stand in a line, one behind the other.*
- *Take a step forward with one leg, placing the ball of your foot on the floor first and then slowly pressing the heel to the floor.*
- *Take another step forward with the other leg, again placing the ball of your foot on the floor first and the heel last.*
- *Camel-walk for a few more steps.*

Camels have thick fur to protect them against the sandstorms that blow in the desert. When the wind blows hard, camels close their nostrils and use an extra eyelid and two sets of eyelashes to protect their eyes from the sand.

Sand Storm

Have the children pretend they're camels in a sandstorm.

- *Try to close your nostrils without using your hands.*
- *Lower your eyelids and eyelashes by looking at the tip of your nose.*
- *Feel the wind swirling at your feet.*
- *Feel the gritty sand blowing all over your face, chest, arms, and legs.*

55 **Sitting Still**

Read the following instructions out loud:

- *Sit on your knees with your body upright and your hands on your buttocks.*
- *Bend your head backward and arch your back.*
- *Hold this position as long as it is comfortable.*
- *Now sit up again.*

Play the game one or two more times.

❖ ❖ ❖ ❖ ❖ ❖ **Camels lie down to rest.** ❖ ❖ ❖ ❖ ❖ ❖

❖ ❖ ❖ ❖ ❖ ❖ **Next we come to the meerkat exhibit.**
"Meerkat" means "marsh cat," but it is
not a cat nor does it live in a marsh. It is a
type of mongoose that lives in the desert. ❖ ❖ ❖ ❖ ❖ ❖

Meerkat

Meerkats have long, skinny bodies, short legs, and poor vision. Only six inches high when they stand on four legs, they are twice as tall when they stand on two legs.

 Hunting Party

56

Tell the children: *The mob that hunts together, stays together—but meerkats usually eat alone. Are you hungry?*

- *Stand on your haunches, with your feet on the floor and your bottom on your heels.*
- *Pop up quickly and stand up straight.*
- *Stretch up on tiptoes.*
- *Bob your head up and down while you look around to make sure there are no predators nearby.*
- *Lie on your tummy with your arms beside your body and put your forearms flat on the floor.*
- *Get on your knees and lift your body a little bit up from the floor.*
- *Crawl around the "desert" looking for food.*
- *When you hear the "leader" make a yipping sound to signal he's found food, gather in a circle around the ant hill.*
- *Stand up on tiptoes and bob your head up and down to celebrate the successful hunt!*

Tip: You can act as the "leader" of the "mob," or you can assign that task to one of the children.

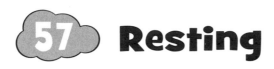

57 **Resting**

Guide the children as follows: *It's time to pile up for a nap.*

- *Lie on your tummy with your arms beside your body.*
- *Put your forearms flat on the floor.*
- *Get on your knees and lift your body a little bit up from the floor.*
- *Crawl to the "sleeping den."*
- *Lie down on the other meerkats, so that everyone is leaning against or laying their heads on someone.*
- *Close your eyes and rest quietly.*

Note: Before playing this game, make sure this amount of physical contact is permitted in your setting. Adjust the amount of contact in the game as needed.

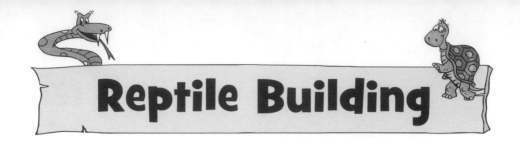

Reptile Building

Your adventure in the zoo continues.
You arrive at the reptile house,
where the cold-blooded animals live.
The first reptile you see is a
crocodile, sunning itself on a rock.

Crocodile

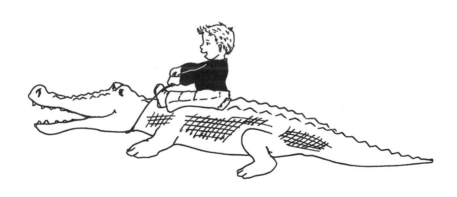

A croc might look like it's lazy,
but it can move fast on dry land
and even faster in water.

Wiggle-Waggle

Teach the children to belly-crawl like a crocodile:

- *Lie face down on the floor.*
- *Press your legs together and stretch your toes to make your "tail."*
- *Bend your elbows and put your hands flat on the floor next to your chest.*
- *Raise your body up slowly by extending your arms.*
- *Use your hands to walk around in search of your prey, dragging your tail behind you. As you wiggle-waggle across the floor, say this rhyme:*

> *The crocodile lies in the water (crocodile posture),*
>
> *The crocodile lies still (stay still and quiet),*
>
> *The crocodile comes near (creep forward),*
>
> *Oops!…He bites you on your rear*
> *(stretch your hands forward like a big*
> *mouth and make it open and close).*

You now stand in front of the snake enclosure and watch them slither around.

Snake

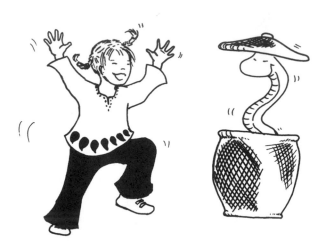

❖ ❖ ❖ ❖ ❖ ❖ **Have you heard of snake charmers who can make snakes dance by moving their own bodies and flutes?** ❖ ❖ ❖ ❖ ❖ ❖

59 Snake Charmer

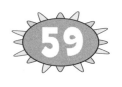

any size

Music: Flute

Instruct the children as follows:

- *Lie on your tummy.*
- *As soon as you see the flute being played, raise your body and sit on your heels.*

- *Move your body around in a slow, rhymic motion.*
- *When the music stops, stop moving, lie down on your tummy again, and stay very still.*

Snakes are remarkable for their long, slender, limbless bodies. They move very fluidly.

 # Hissing

Read the instruction below out loud:

- *Lie on your tummy.*
- *Press your legs together.*
- *Put your hands flat on the floor next to your chest.*
- *Push with your arms and raise your chest up from the floor.*
- *"Hissssss" like a snake.*
- *Lower your body to the floor.*
- *Lift, hiss, and lower one or two more times.*

A little farther along you can look through the glass and watch the frogs jumping.

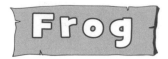

Frog

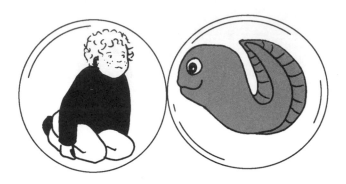

❖ ❖ ❖ ❖ ❖ ❖ ❖ **Before a frog becomes a frog,**
it is first a frogspawn (egg)
and then a tadpole. ❖ ❖ ❖ ❖ ❖ ❖ ❖

61 Frogspawn

Say: *Imagine you are inside an egg filled with jelly, where you will slowly evolve into a tadpole.*

- *Sit on your knees and bring your head down to the floor.*
- *Make yourself as small as you can.*
- *Feel yourself floating in the jiggly jelly—slowly growing leg and arm nubs and patiently waiting to grow into a tadpole.*

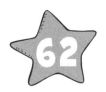

62 Tadpole

Tell the children: *Slowly you change into a tadpole.*

- *Lie on your tummy.*
- *Bend your arms at the elbows and bend your legs at the knees so that your hands and feet are close to your body.*
- *Stretch your legs out straight.*
- *Press your legs together and point your toes. Now you are a tadpole with a long tail.*
- *Keep your arms bent at the elbows and close to your body, with your hands near your shoulders.*
- *Swim around the pond by sliding your tail from side to side and paddling with your hands.*

63 Sprouting Limbs

Have the children change from tadpoles into frogs.

- *Feel your tail disappear and your back legs begin to appear as you slowly spread your legs.*
- *Feel your separated tail grow into two strong legs as you bend them at the knees.*
- *Feel your front legs appear as you move your hands away from your body.*

Hopping and Croaking

any
size

Say to the children: *Now you are a real frog, ready to hop and sing for joy!*

- *Sit on your haunches with your feet flat on the floor, your knees apart, and your bottom on your heels.*
- *Put your hands flat on the floor in front of you.*
- *Breathe in and jump up so that both your feet leave the floor at the same time.*
- *Breathe out as you come back down.*
- *Hop around the pond a few more times as you sing this song:*

> *Ga-gung! went the little green frog one day,*
> *Ga-gung! went the little green frog.*
> *Ga-gung! went the little green frog one day,*
> *Ga-gung, ga-gung, ga-gung!*

**In the next pond,
you see a variety of turtles—
big ones and little ones,
green ones and brown ones,
spotted ones and striped ones.**

Turtle

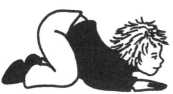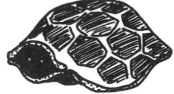

Turtles pull their heads back into their shells when they don't feel safe.

65 Sliding into My Shell

Ask the children to try sliding in and out of their shell like a turtle.

- *Sit up straight and stretch your legs out in front of you, spread apart.*
- *As you breathe in, raise your arms above your head.*
- *As you breathe out, bend forward and bring your arms and head to the floor.*
- *Slide your arms backward to rest against your thighs with your palms facing upwards.*
- *Close your eyes and remain still in this position.*
- *Slowly straighten up again.*

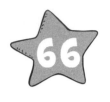

Hare and Tortoise

Create your own instructions to teach the children how to play the following game:

- Talk about the differences in speed between a hare and a tortoise.
- Ask each child whether they like to go fast or slow.
- Divide the children into two groups: "hares" and "tortoises."
- All the children stand on one side of the room, side by side.
- When you call out "hares," all the children belonging to that group run quickly to the other side of the room.
- When you call out "tortoises," all the children belonging to that group cross to the other side of the room very slowly.

Tip: You can have the children switch roles and play the game again. As a variation, you can tell the children to move in a different way— for example, walk, crawl, waggle, shuffle, hop, limp, walk backward, skate, etc.

Chameleon

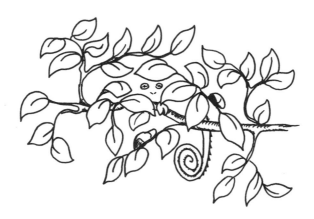

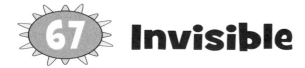 **You come to a glass case filled with plants. It looks like no animals are living in there, but if you look carefully you will see the chameleon. He is very hard to see, because he turns into the same color as the leaf he is sitting on, the branch he is walking along, or the rock he is hiding under.**

67 Invisible

Ask the children the following questions:

Would you sometimes like to be invisible? If so, when?

Is it possible to be nearly invisible sometimes? How?

**A chameleon's tongue is as long
as its body and tail put together.
He has to keep it rolled up in his mouth.
If he wants to catch his prey,
he can shoot out his tongue
and bring it back to his mouth
again as fast as lightning.**

 # Darting Tongue

any
size

Guide the children as follows:

- *Stand up straight.*
- *Quickly stick out your tongue.*
- *Quickly suck your tongue back into your mouth.*
- *Quickly stick out your tongue and suck it back in a few times while you breathe in and out through your mouth.*
- *Feel how cold the breath is when it comes in through your tongue.*

Tip: This game is easier for children who can roll their tongues inward into a shape like a straw, but some children are genetically unable to do so.

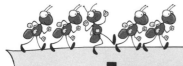

Insect House

Now we've arrived at the insect house,
where the flying and crawling bugs
are kept in glass enclosures.

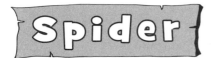

Spider

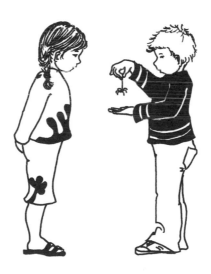

Have you ever felt
the tickling of a little spider
as it walks over your body?

69 Tickle-Tickle!

Divide the children into pairs and read the following instructions aloud:

- *Decide who will be the "spider" and who will be the "kid."*
- *Sit one behind the other, with the spider in back and the kid in front.*
- *If you're the spider, make a spider out of your hands and crawl up and down up your partner's back as you both sing this song:*

> *The itsy-bitsy spider went up the water spout,*
>
> *Down came the rain and washed the spider out,*
>
> *Out came the sun and dried up all the rain,*
>
> *Then the itsy-bitsy spider went up the spout again.*

Have the children change places and play the game again.

Tip: While the "spiders" are crawling up and down the other kids' backs, the kids sitting in front can do hand gestures for "sun" and "rain." This will make the game even more interactive and fun for all the children.

Next to the spiders you discover beetles of many colors, shapes, and sizes. The first one you see is a ladybug with lovely red wings with seven black dots.

Ladybug

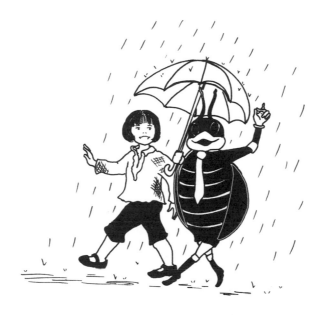

Ladybugs like rain, because it makes the plants grow and plants attract aphids, which ladybugs love to eat.

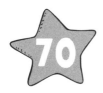 **70** # Rain Dance

Say:

- *Stand up straight. Leave enough space between you and your friends so that you won't bump into each other when you start dancing.*

- *Act out the movements as you sing this song:*

Put up your umbrella
When the rain comes down.
Wear a happy smile
And wipe away a frown.
Splash in all the puddles
And do a little dance.
Rain is just the thing we need
For Miss Ladybug's spring plants.

Tip: You can make up a melody or borrow one from a popular children's song.

Some beetles even eat caterpillars, so it's a good thing the caterpillars have their own house, well out of harm's way.

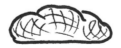

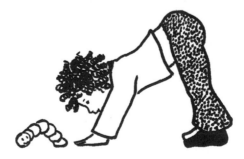

**Before a butterfly becomes a butterfly.
it has had a whole life as a caterpillar.**

 # 71 Creeping

Instruct the children as follows:

- *Stand up straight with your feet apart.*
- *Bend forward at your waist and lower your upper body until you are facing your knees.*
- *Put your hands flat on the floor in front of you.*
- *Scoot your feet forward a little bit.*
- *Scoot your hands forward a little bit and then scoot your feet forward a little bit.*
- *Creep around like that as you look for a nice juicy leaf to munch. When your tummy is full, you are ready for your transformation.*

**Caterpillars wrap themselves in a cocoon.
where they sleep and transform into
a moth or a beautiful butterfly.**

 # 72 Cocoon

Say to the children: *Make yourself very small and imagine you are in your cocoon.*

- *Sit with your bottom on your heels.*

- *Lean forward slowly.*
- *Place your head on the floor and your arms alongside your body.*
- *Keep very still while your transformation is happening.*
- *Feel your caterpillar self slowly changing into a beautiful butterfly.*

Butterfly

Butterflies need the warmth of the sun in order to fly. They often sit on a tree or a wall and spread open their wings so that the sun can warm them.

73 Sunbathing

Tell the children that they should now let the sun warm them up:

- *Lie on the floor with your "wings" (arms and legs) spread out.*
- *Close your eyes.*
- *Imagine you are lying on a flower with the sun shining on you.*
- *Can you feel the warmth? Do you feel ready to fly?*

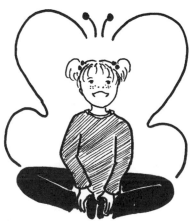

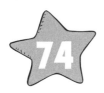 **74** # Flower Power

Props: Paper, plastic, or cloth butterflies on sticks, for about half of the children

Say: *Now the butterfly is ready to fly around in search of flowers from which to sip nectar.*

Divide the children into two groups: "butterflies" and "flowers." Tell the "flowers" to scatter themselves around the room and give every "butterfly" a butterfly attached to a stick. Then say:

- *The "flowers" should stand tall like a flower in bloom and close their eyes.*

- *The "butterflies" should move around the room, fluttering their wings, looking for a "flower" on which to land. Only one butterfly at a time can rest on a flower.*

- *A "butterfly" settles on an open "flower" by gently resting the paper butterfly on a part of the other child's body.*

- *The "flower" then says aloud the name of the body part on which the "butterfly" has landed.*

- *If the "flower" guesses correctly, the "butterfly" can continue flying and settle on other flowers.*

- *After a while, the children change places and play the game again.*

Tip: You can purchase paper, plastic, or cloth butterflies on sticks at various garden, hobby, and gift stores or you can make them yourself.

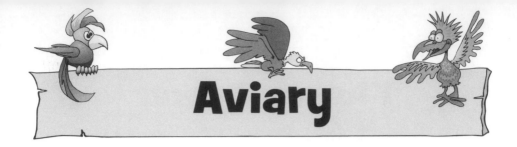

Aviary

Your journey through the zoo brings you to several large cages, where you see a variety of birds.

Parrot

The parrots are sitting in a tree. You can recognize them by their large heads, short necks, and curved beaks. Many have colored feathers and "masks" around their eyes. Parrots show their feelings by making the pupils of their eyes larger or smaller. Small pupils usually mean the parrot is angry or upset, often when he is ready to bite. However, it can also mean he is excited about something he likes.

75 Angry Eyes, Happy Eyes

any size

Tell the children to show how they feel using only their eyes.

76

Flying

Props: Two colored scarves for each child

Tie a scarf around each wrist of each child and then say:
Now you have big colored wings with which to fly.

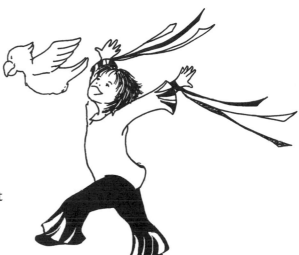

- *Spread your "wings" and flap them up and down.*

- *Now fly around the room—soaring high by getting on tiptoes and swooping low by bending your knees.*

Tip: If you're working with several children, you might want to have another adult help you tie and untie the scarves.

77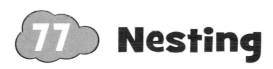

Nesting

Teach the children how to play the game as follows:

- The children act out the movements as they say this rhyme:

  Penelope Parrot up high in the tree,

  Will you come down and play with me?

  We'll fly and dance and feather your nest,

  Then we'll PLOP onto your perch for a nice little rest.

- On the word "plop," they drop to the floor, lie down, close their eyes, and rest.

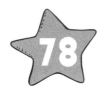

Fluffy Feathers

Props: A feather for each child, in a range of colors, scattered around the floor

Divide the group into pairs and guide the children as follows:

- *Pick up a feather from the floor.*
- *Stroke your face and arms with the feather.*
- *Stroke your friend's face and arms with the feather.*
- *What differences do you feel when you do it and when someone else does it?*
- *Throw the feather into the air and see if you can keep it up by blowing it.*
- *Now pretend that you are a feather and drift around the room.*

❖ ❖ ❖ ❖ ❖ ❖ **Behind the parrot enclosure**
you can see the flamingos standing
in the pond. They search for food
by scooping their beaks through the
water, sort of like a fishing net. ❖ ❖ ❖ ❖ ❖ ❖

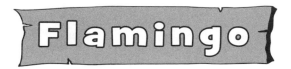
Flamingo

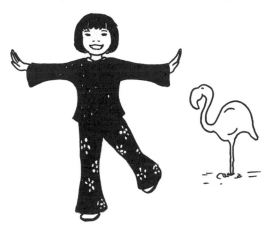

✣ ✤ ✣ ✤ ✣ **When flamingos rest,**
they often stand on one leg. ✣ ✤ ✣ ✤ ✣ ✤ ✣

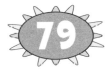

(79) Standing on One Leg

any size

Ask the children: *How long can you stand on one leg?*

- *Stand up straight with your arms by your sides.*
- *Bring your arms up until they are level with your shoulders.*
- *Lift your right foot up behind you.*
- *Stand on one foot as still and as long as you can.*
- *Do it again with your left leg.*

✣ ✤ ✣ ✤ ✣ ✤ **Flamingos do a special dance to impress each**
other. The whole group often dances together
so they'll all lay eggs at the same time. ✣ ✤ ✣ ✤ ✣ ✤

Flamingo Dance

Music: Salsa or any other kind of dance music

Do the flamingo dance together three times:

- *Stand side-by-side in a line.*
- *Tilt your "beak" (nose) up at the sky and wag it back and forth.*
- *Spread your "wings" (arms) out wide on either side.*
- *Take two sideways steps to the right.*
- *Take two sideways steps to the left.*
- *Shuffle around in a circle.*
- *Put your "wings" (arms) behind your back and take a bow.*

Peacock

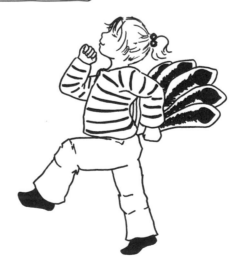

Peacocks show off their beautiful tail feathers, which have all the colors of the rainbow. They show their fancy feathers not only for pea hens but also for other animals and people.

 # Showing Off any size

Tell the children to show off their back side and strut around the room proudly.

The peacock makes a sound like "may-awe, may-awe!"

 # Bird Call any size

Have the children try to make a peacock call.

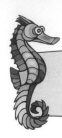

Aquarium

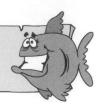

Now you have reached the aquarium, where hundreds of colored fish welcome you. In the tanks that house the reef creatures, you see corals, mussels, oysters, sponges, sea anemones, sea urchins, crabs, lobsters, sea cucumbers, and starfish.

Starfish

A starfish has five arms, a head in the center of its body, and a mouth underneath. Did you know that if a starfish loses an arm, a new one grows in its place?

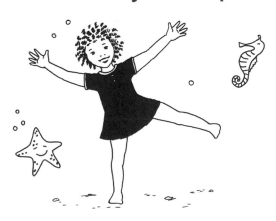

 # Twinkle, Twinkle, Little Starfish

any
size

Say: *Pretend you are a starfish that grows four new points.*

- *Lie down.*
- *Bring your legs together and put your arms next to your sides.*
- *Spread your arms and legs out as far as you can, like a huge starfish.*
- *Bring your legs together and your arms to your sides again.*
- *Make yourself into a starfish a few more times.*

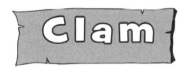
Clam

Clams have a soft body that is protected by a hard shell made of calcium. The shell opens only when it's time for the clam to eat.

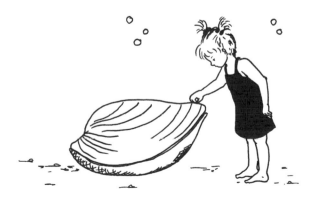

Open and Shut

Tell the children: *Act as if you are a hungry clam.*

- *Sit up straight with your legs out in front of you.*
- *Bend forward and bring your face to your knees.*
- *Hold your toes or your ankles.*
- *Open your "shell" by slowly straightening up.*
- *Stretch your arms above your head.*
- *Open and close your shell a few more times.*

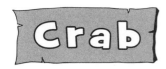

Crabs can move in all directions— including sideways—which comes in quite handy both in the water and on land.

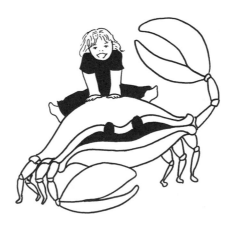

85 Crab Walk

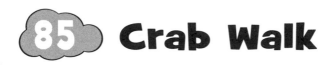

Say to the children: *Try walking sideways like a crab.*

- *Sit on the floor with your legs stretched out in front of you.*
- *Put your hands flat on the floor behind you, fingers pointing forward.*
- *Lean backward and then lift your body off the ground.*
- *Walk sideways on your hands and feet a few steps to your right.*
- *Walk sideways to the left.*
- *Walk sideways to the right and then to the left a few more times.*

After you leave the reef exhibit, you go down to the big tanks where the animals who live in the depths of the ocean swim about. Beware! A shark may suddenly sneak up on you!

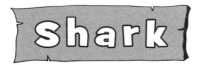

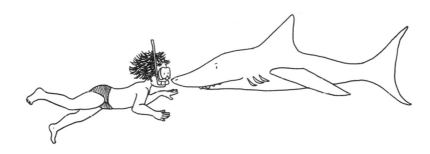

Sharks move forward by swinging their tails back and forth. They use their two pelvic fins and two pectoral fins to steer and stop.

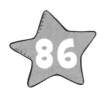 # **86** **Prowling**

Teach the children this exercise by saying the following:
Make yourself feel as strong as a shark and swim after your prey.

- *Lie on your tummy.*
- *Bend your legs up and point your toes toward the ceiling to make your "tail."*
- *Bring both arms behind you and entwine your fingers together.*
- *Slide your arms up to the middle of your back to make your "fins."*
- *Lift your head and swim like a shark prowling for food in the ocean by moving your tail back and forth and your fins up and down.*

Next we visit the place housing the animals that live in the coldest regions of the earth. Here we find king penguins and sea lions, who spend time both in and out of the water.

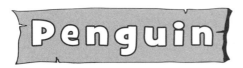

Penguin

Penguins usually walk upright, shuffling along. When they want to go faster, they skid across the ice on their stomachs.

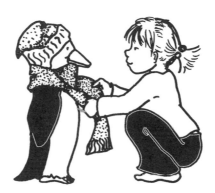

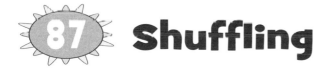

87 ☼ **Shuffling**

Ask the children to try walking like a penguin, using the following instructions:

- *Stand with your legs pressed tightly together.*
- *Press your heels together and slide your toes outward.*
- *Put your arms down at your sides.*
- *Lift your hands up from the wrists, so that your palms are facing the floor.*
- *Shuffle around, taking tiny steps quickly and close together.*

Penguins live only in the southern hemisphere, mostly in areas that are extremely cold and where the land is covered in snow and ice. To keep warm, penguins stand very close together in groups.

Huddling

whole group

Guide the children in how to play the following game:

- The children stand single-file in a line and hold hands with the "penguins" in front and back of them.
- The child at the front of the line stays where she is; this is the "center."
- The child at the back moves to the center, and the other children follow.
- Still holding hands, the children form a tight circle around the center, creating a dense mass of "penguins" standing very close together.
- The group then unwinds into a long line.

When penguins feel cold, they warm themselves by flapping their wings against their sides.

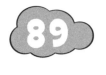 # Chilly Willy Dance

Music: Rhythmic

Teach the children how to play the game as follows:

- The children do the penguin dance to rhythmic music. They shuffle around and flap their wings by slapping their palms on their thighs (see Game #87).
- When the music stops, call out the name of a part of the body—nose, hand, knee, ear, etc.
- The children cluster together and rub that part of the body to "warm it up."
- Do a few rounds, calling out a different body part each time.

Tip: As a variation, rather than calling out body parts, you can call out different postures for the children to take—such as lying down, sitting, kneeling, and squatting.

Penguins do not make nests. When the female lays an egg, the male rolls it onto his feet. They are even able to walk around without dropping the egg.

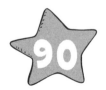 # Precious Cargo

Props: A small rubber ball for each child

Read the following instructions aloud:

- *Stand up straight.*

- *Put a ball between your feet and hold it tight with your ankles.*
- *Walk around the room without dropping the ball.*

When penguin chicks hatch, they sit on the mother's feet. The mother has a fold of skin that protects them, making the little ones feel safe and warm. The mother moves around carrying the baby on her feet.

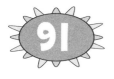 # **Mama and Chick**

Divide the group into pairs. Say: *Can you and your friend walk like mama and baby penguins?*

- *Decide who will be the "mama" and who will be the "chick."*
- *If you're the chick, stand on your mama's feet and hold onto her wings (arms).*
- *If you're the mama, walk around with your chick on your feet.*
- *Change places and play the game again.*

Penguins sleep standing up and often lean against their mothers or partners as they sleep. That way everyone stays nice and warm.

92 # **Feeling** the **Breath**

Divide the group into pairs and instruct the children as follows:

- *Stand back-to-back with your partner.*
- *Be very quiet.*
- *Close your eyes and feel how warm you are when you stand close together.*
- *Can you feel your partner breathing?*

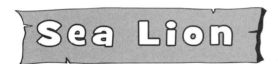

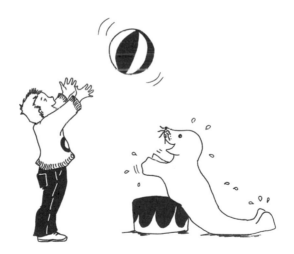

❖ ❖ ❖ ❖ ❖ ❖ **Sea lions can move either on land or in the water, but in the water they move easily and freely.** ❖ ❖ ❖ ❖ ❖ ❖

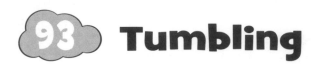

93 Tumbling

Say to the children: *Play in the water and on the ice like a sea lion.*

- *Lie flat on your tummy with your legs pressed together and stretched out.*
- *Lean on your forearms with your arms angled outward (elbows close to body).*
- *Use your arms to pull yourself forward along the floor, dragging your feet behind you.*
- *Raise your arms and legs from the ground and clap your hands and feet together at the same time.*
- *Roll over a few times.*

Sea lions can move across the ice very easily and often climb on the ice floes.

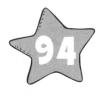 # 94 Sliding

Props: Two pieces of paper for each child

Tell the children to try sliding across the room like a sea lion on an ice floe.

- *Stand barefoot and place each foot on its own piece of paper.*
- *Slide across the room on these ice floes, keeping your feet on the paper.*

Tip: For variation, you can put a piece of paper under each knee and each hand and crawl-slide across the floor. Make sure to have enough sheets of paper.

Nocturnal Animal Enclosure

While you're sleeping at night, some animals are wide awake. These animals are called <u>nocturnal</u>. When it gets dark, they go out in search of food. To see nocturnal animals in the zoo or in the wild, you have to be patient, because most of them are sleeping in a safe hiding place.

Owl
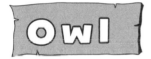

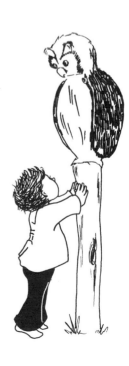

The owl leaves his roost at night to go hunting. He can see very well in the dark with those great big eyes, and his hearing is excellent. He can see enough by the light of the moon and stars to search for his prey, and in complete darkness he can hear a mouse scuttling along from far away.

Scouting

Ask the children: *What do you see in the dark of night?*

- *Squat on your haunches with your legs together and your feet on the floor.*
- *Bring your arms behind you and lock your fingers together.*
- *Open your eyes wide and look over your shoulder as far as you can, like an owl looking for prey.*
- *Face forward again and look all around you.*
- *Spread your "wings" (arms) wide.*
- *"Fly" around the room and hoot like an owl.*

 # Guess Who-oo-oo?

Teach the children how to play the game as follows:

- The group sits together facing the leader and closes their eyes.
- One child is tagged (by the leader) and stands in front of the group.
- Hold a big sheet in front of the child so the others can't see who it is—and leave only his feet visible.
- Ask the children to open their eyes and guess who is behind the sheet (without looking around at the other players to see who might be missing).
- Play the game a few times, each time tagging a different child and showing a different part of the body (for example, covering all but the child's hair or all but an elbow).

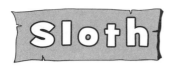

Sloth

A sloth spends most of its life hanging upside down from tree branches. It can bend its head straight back so that it doesn't always have to look at the world upside down.

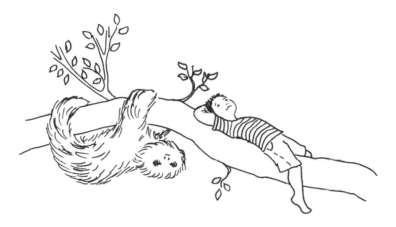

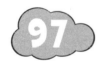 **Slow Motion**

Read the following instruction aloud to the children:

- *Lie on your tummy.*
- *Put your hands and toes on the floor.*
- *Lift your left foot and right hand from the floor. Move them forward very slowly and place them down on the floor.*
- *Do the same with your right foot and left hand, dragging your body forward deliberately.*
- *Take a few more slow-as-a-sloth steps.*
- *Look through your legs. How does the world look from upside down?*

Goodbye, Zoo

✺ ✺ ✺ ✺ ✺ ✺ **We've had a wonderful zoo adventure. Now it's time to go home.** ✺ ✺ ✺ ✺ ✺ ✺

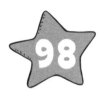 # Animal Song

Say: *Let's sing about the animals as we walk to the bus station.*

- *Stand up straight.*
- *As you walk, sing this song and make the movements that go with it:*

    They can say what they want, but the elephant
    Has the biggest bottom (slap your bottom),
    And the giraffe has the longest neck (stretch your neck),
    And the hippo has the biggest mouth (open your mouth wide).

Tip: The children can either walk in place or walk around the room.

✺ ✺ ✺ ✺ ✺ ✺ **We arrive at the bus station, where the bus is waiting to take us home.** ✺ ✺ ✺ ✺ ✺ ✺

Riding Home

Guide the children as follows:

- *Sit on the floor in a row, one passenger behind another, with your legs stretched out in front of you.*

- *Bring your hands in front of you and point your elbows outward.*

- *Make circles with each of your arms in a forward direction, like the wheels on the bus, going round and round.*

- *At the same time, scoot your bottom back and forth a little. The bus is now moving forward.*

- *While you ride along in the bus, sing this song:*

> *The wheels on the bus go round and round,*
> *Round and round, round and round.*
> *The wheels on the bus go round and round,*
> *All through the town.*

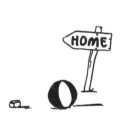 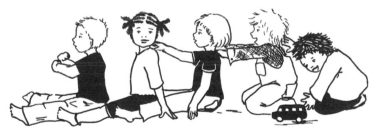

Settle Down

Your exciting zoo adventure is over, and you have reached home safe and sound. In the evening, you get ready for a good night's sleep.

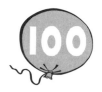 ## 100 Sleepy Dance

any size

Have the children sing this song and make the movements that go with it (see the top of the next page):

1. I can't do any more, I am so tired
(stand with knees bent slightly and arms hanging down loosely).

2. I stretch myself up to the stars
(stand up straight with hands stretched above head).

3. I relax in the moonlight
(spread arms and lower to shoulder-level to make an arc like a half-moon).

4. I get undressed
(bend down and pretend to take off your pants and then your shirt).

5. I get dressed for bed
(pretend to put on pajamas).

6. I look for my stuffed animals
(look left and then right).

7. I pick up my rabbit
(bend sideways to the left).
I pick up my teddy bear
(bend sideways to the right).

8. I stand up tall and say "good night."

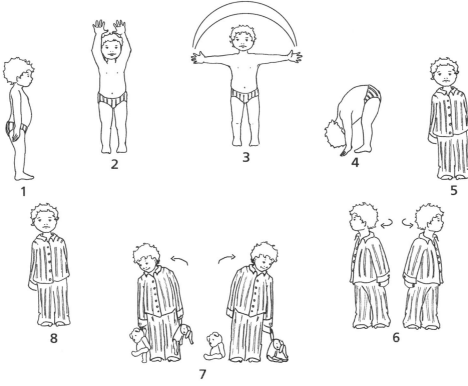

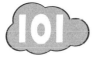

101 Brushing Teeth

any size

Instruct the children as follows:

- *Move your toothbrush (index finger) back and forth in front of your mouth.*
- *Pretend to take a mouthful of water and fill up your cheeks with it.*
- *Spit the water into the sink.*
- *Show your nice, clean teeth to your friends and give a broad grin.*

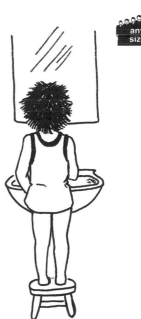

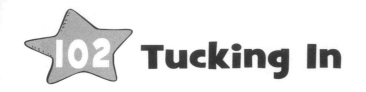

102 Tucking In

Teach the children how to play the game as follows:

- The children sit up straight and hold one hand in front of them with all the fingers standing up—still awake. As they "tuck in" their fingers, they say this rhyme, decreasing the number of fingers standing by one finger each time:

Five little fingers standing on the bed,

One fell off and bumped his head,

Mama called the doctor, and the doctor said,

"That's what you get for standing on the bed."

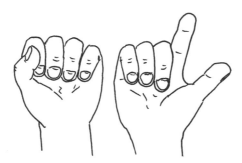

- The children tuck in the fingers on their other hand, one by one, as they say the rhyme again.
- Then they all say, "Now all ten fingers are tucked into bed!"

Tip: If any fingers are "naughty" and won't lie down, the children can push them down with their other hand.

Sleeping

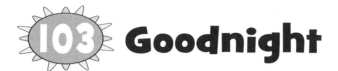

103 Goodnight

Say to the children:

- *Lie down.*
- *Close your eyes and let your body slowly melt into the floor.*
- *Be still and quiet.*
- *Stretch your neck out like a giraffe.*
- *Spread your arms and legs like a starfish.*
- *Lie on your side like a sea lion.*
- *Draw your knees up to your chest like a fox.*

104 Dream Time

Tell the children the following: *The zoo animals visit you in your dreams.*

- *Lie on your back with your arms at your sides.*
- *Close your eyes.*
- *Think about the animals you met on your zoo adventure today.*
- *Hear the elephant trumpeting, "It was great to see you."*
- *Hear the snake hiss, "Until next time."*
- *Hear the parrot squawk, "Good night!"*
- *Hear the bear growl, "Sleep well."*

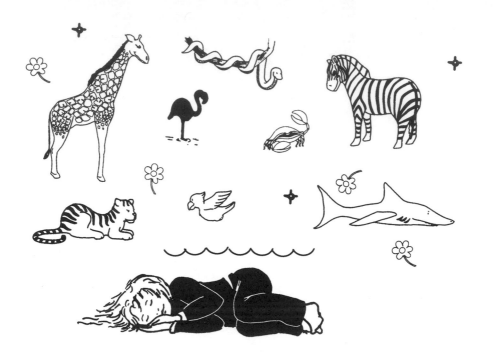

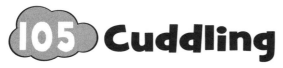 Cuddling

Props: A small stuffed animal for each child

Guide the children through this game by saying the following:

- *Lie on your back.*
- *Close your eyes.*
- *Hold your stuffed animal close to your tummy.*
- *Wiggle your fingers and toes.*
- *Open your eyes and look at your tummy.*
- *Try moving the stuffed animal with your breathing.*

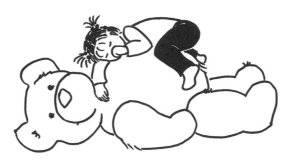

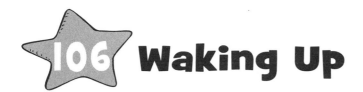

106 Waking Up

Say:

- *Open your eyes.*
- *Stretch out like a giraffe.*
- *Roll back and forth like a crocodile.*
- *Sit up with a straight back like an ape.*
- *Get up on your hands and knees like a zebra.*
- *Stand up slowly and stretch your neck like a flamingo.*
- *Think about your zoo adventure and smile.*
- *See you on the next adventure!*

Animal Fables

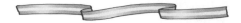

Animal fables are a delightful and effective way to teach life lessons, social norms, and values to children. A fable is a ficticious short story in which animals, legendary figures, or mythical beings act out realistic situations in order to reveal a moral. Fables have been used in all cultures for centuries as a way of writing about human life.

In animal fables, the animals think, feel, act, and talk like humans. Young children are fond of and fascinated with animals, and they are influenced by how animal characters behave and the consequences of those behaviors in stories. Animal fables can help children learn how to handle challenges and how to "do the right thing." For example, a fable might show that mistakes can result from being too stubborn and that problems can be solved by being open-minded.

Animal fables are a good way to help children understand the ideas behind yoga life rules. Stories that are linked to the sounds and movements an animal makes can also stimulate the children's imaginations.

You can read a fable about a specific animal to the children before you begin the games that are based on that animal. Another option is to read a fable before or after class. At home, the fables can be read during quiet play time or at bedtime. After reading a story, you can discuss its meaning and message with the children. The stories and discussions offer the children an effortless and enjoyable way of thinking about good and bad in the world.

Discussion

- Introduce the children to the term "fable," explaining that it is a story in which animals act like people in order to teach a life lesson.

- After reading the story, discuss it with the children. To stimulate the discussion, you might ask the children questions, such as:
  - Do you know the animals in this story?
  - What did you like about the story, and how did it make you feel?
  - Was it a happy or a sad story, and how did you feel about it?

- Did the story have a happy ending?
- Who are the main characters in the story?
- Which character did you find the most important, the silliest, the stupidest, the nicest, etc.?
- Who did you like in the story? Who did you not like?
- Did strange things happen in the story? What did you find strange and why?
- If you had been able to take part in the story, what would you have done?
- What do you think is the moral, or lesson, of the story?

Tip: You can use a glove puppet to ask the questions. If time allows, the children can act out the story or a part of the story. Then encourage the children to talk about how they felt.

The Stories

Elephant Eats Out

One day Elephant was very hungry. He went into a restaurant and sat down at a table. "Waiter!" called Elephant, "I want lentil soup, carrots, and fried potatoes. And hurry up about it, because I'm very, very hungry." After a short time, the waiter came back with the food. Elephant looked at his plate crossly. "You call this a meal?" he complained. "You've given me much too little. A bird couldn't live on this. I want a bathtub of soup, a bucket of carrots, and a mountain of potatoes." The waiter went back to the kitchen and came back with a mountain of food for Elephant. "Yes! That's what I wanted," said Elephant. Elephant finished every crumb in just a few mouthfuls. "Delicious!" said Elephant as he wiped his mouth with his napkin. He had eaten until his stomach had blown up like a balloon. Now he wanted to go home, but when he tried to stand up, he couldn't move. His stomach was so fat he was stuck between the chair and the table. When he tried to stand up, the chair clung to his backside. When he tried to push himself away from the table, the table stayed clamped on his stomach. He pushed and pulled, but it didn't help at all. He was stuck in his chair! It grew later and later. All the other guests went home. The cooks took off their aprons and started cleaning up. The waiters turned out the lights, and they all went home. Elephant sat there all by himself. Once in a while, he let out a big burp. As the sky grew darker and darker, Elephant sat alone, stuck in the chair, thinking, "Maybe I shouldn't have eaten so much."

Mrs. Rhino

Mrs. Rhino wanted a new dress. She went to the shop, where in the window she spotted a lovely pink dress with red flowers on it. The dress was made of lace and decorated with gold ribbons. She went into the shop and tried on the dress. She looked in the mirror and said to the assistant, "I don't think it really suits me." "Oh, but madam," said the assistant, "you look wonderful in that dress. When you wear it, everyone will admire you and smile at you." Mrs. Rhino looked at herself in the mirror again. Yes, maybe the assistant was right. "I'll take the dress, and I'll keep it on." Mrs. Rhino paid for the dress and left the shop. Everyone who saw her froze and stared. Some people laughed. Some shook their heads or wrinkled their foreheads. Mrs. Rhino enjoyed all this attention, and with every step she felt more and more beautiful. She walked proudly down the street—pink lace, red flowers, gold ribbons, and all.

Lion and Beetle

One day King Lion looked in the mirror. "What a wonderful animal I am! How strong I am," he said to himself. He put on his royal cloak and his crown, and hung his medals around his neck so everyone could see he was king. He went out for a kingly stroll, and everyone who saw him bowed deeply. Lion felt he deserved such special treatment, because he was strong and fine. As he walked down the road he came across a lowly little beetle. Did the beetle bow to him? Lion didn't think so, and he boomed out, "Beetle, I order you to bow deeply before me!" "Your majesty," answered the beetle, "I am bowing. If you look at me carefully, you will see that." Lion bent down. "Beetle," he said, "I can hardly see you down there. I'm not really sure you are bowing to me." Lion leaned lower and lower. The heavy crown and all those medals weighed him down so much that he fell right over and bumped his head. He growled and rolled into a ditch at the side of the road. Beetle got the shock of his life and ran off. And Lion? King Lion? He was nowhere to be seen. He was covered in mud from top to toe.

Tiger and the Wishing Tree

There once was a poor young man who had no possessions except what he was wearing. He went in search of the wishing tree, the tree that granted all wishes. After a little while, he found the tree. *From now on life would be good,* he thought with certainty, *a life without problems.* He looked at the tree and touched the trunk and said to himself, "How wonderful it would be to have a big bag full of gold." At that moment a pile of gold appeared in front of him. Speechless with happiness, he wished for a chest full of jewels. No sooner had he thought the wish than a chest overflowing with precious stones appeared at his feet. He became very excited and shouted, "I want a palace made of gold!" And there before him sparkled the golden palace. He felt hungry from his long journey, so he wished for a good meal. In the blink of an eye, a big table with the most delicious dishes stood in front of him. He ate and ate until he could eat no more. Then he was tired, and the only thing he wanted was a lovely soft bed to rest in. Suddenly, a golden bed with a goose-feather mattress and a feather pillow appeared. He lay down on his beautiful bed and imagined that he was in the middle of the forest where tigers lived. He imagined that a tiger might come and jump on him and eat him up. Sure enough, along came a tiger, who pounced on him and ate him up.

Bear and Crow

One day Bear went off to the city. He put on his best clothes, with a handsome hat and shiny new shoes. "How good I look," Bear said to himself. "I am sure to impress everyone who sees me." Crow was eavesdropping and heard every word Bear had said. "I'm sorry to disappoint you, but your clothes are not beautiful at all," said Crow. "I come from the city, and the men there don't wear hats; they wear a pan on their heads. Instead of shoes they wear paper bags on their feet." "Oh, how stupid of me!" said Bear, "I am wearing quite the wrong clothes for the city!" Quickly he ran home and put a pan on his head and paper bags on his feet. Then he set off for the city. When Bear arrived in the city, everyone pointed at him and laughed. "What a stupid bear!" they said. Bear was very embarrassed and went home again. On the way he saw Crow again. "Crow, you tricked me!" "I told you everything," said Crow, as he flew off, "but I never said I was speaking the truth." Even though Crow was high up in the sky, Bear could still hear him laughing.

Fox and the Duck Sisters

Daisy Duck and her sister Dahlia Duck were waddling along to the pond for their morning swim. Every morning they waddled along the same path to the same pond, so they knew the way quite well. One morning they met Fox, who was sitting on a tree stump at the side of the path. "Good morning, ladies," said Fox. "Where is your journey taking you today?" "Quack, quack, quack," said the Duck Sisters. "We are going to the pond for our morning swim. Quack, quack, quack. We come along here every morning." Fox smiled and slyly showed his great big teeth. When the sun rose next morning, Daisy said, "Let's take a different path this morning. I'm a little afraid of Fox. He has such big teeth." Dahlia said, "Don't be silly. Fox was smiling at us so friendly, and I thought he was a real gentleman." The Duck Sisters waddled along their usual path to the pond. There was Fox. He was sitting on the tree stump again but this time he had a big sack with him. "Good morning, ladies," said Fox. "I am so happy to see you again." Dahlia said, "Quack quack, quack. You see, Sister, he is a real gentleman." But Fox opened up his sack and made a leap toward them. The sisters quacked and shrieked. They flapped their wings and snapped their beaks. They flew home and locked the door. The next morning they did not go to the pond. They stayed home and recovered from the shock. "Quack, quack, quack," they said nervously every now and then. The next morning they very carefully went out and found a new way to the pond.

Gorilla and Chimpanzee
Every day Gorilla went walking in the jungle. On the way he met Chimpanzee. Chimpanzee said, "How strange that you are holding an umbrella above your head on a lovely, sunny day like this." "Yes, I don't really want it either," said Gorilla. "I can't enjoy the sun, because the umbrella blocks the sun's rays, but I can't close it. I don't want to leave it behind, because you never know when it might rain." Chimpanzee said, "All you have to do is to cut a few holes in the umbrella, then the sun can shine through them." Gorilla thought this was a very clever idea. He ran home and took his biggest scissors and cut great big holes in his umbrella. Then he went back out to enjoy his walk. How wonderful to feel the sun on his body! But suddenly the sun disappeared behind some clouds and a couple of great big raindrops fell. Then the heavens opened and the rain poured down. Of course, the rain streamed through all the holes in Gorilla's umbrella and he got soaking wet!

Dancing Camel
Camel loved to dance and wanted nothing more than to become a ballerina. She wanted to make every movement graceful and beautiful. Every day she practiced her dance exercises and danced in circles in the hot desert sun. In spite of the blisters on her feet, the pain in her body, and her tiredness, she did not want to stop dancing. One day she decided

that at last she was a good enough dancer, and she invited all the other camels to come and watch her perform. At the end she gave a deep bow and waited for the applause. But none of the camels clapped. One of them stood up and said, "You are a dancing frump, not a ballerina. You'll never be a dancer, because you are just a camel!" Laughing, all the camels left and walked back into the desert. "They don't understand," said the dancer. "I worked so hard to become a good dancer. I am not going to give it up. I will go on dancing, just for myself." That is just what she did, and she enjoyed it enormously.

Crocodile's Wallpaper

Mr. Crocodile loved to lie in bed. The wallpaper in his bedroom was decorated with neat rows of flowers in pretty colors and tidy rows of trees. He looked happily at the wallpaper for hours on end. Mrs. Crocodile could not understand this at all. Why didn't her husband go for a nice walk in the woods, in the fresh air and warm sunshine? "Why don't you come along?" she said. "It's so beautiful and it smells so good." One day he finally decided to go and take a look in the woods. He put on his sunglasses to protect his eyes from the bright sunlight. "Can you see these beautiful plants and flowers," asked his wife. "Don't they smell wonderful?" But Mr. Crocodile was very uncomfortable. "Everything is all higgledy-piggledy; it's such a mess. You can't see what's what because it's all mixed together." Mr. Crocodile fled back to his bedroom. "Phew!" he said, looking at the wallpaper, "these flowers and trees are all nicely in line. I feel quite safe here." From then on Mr. Crocodile hardly ever left his room. He just sat there smiling broadly, looking at the wallpaper. He started to change color, becoming greener and greener. Not a nice brownish crocodile green, but more of a really icky green.

Mouse and the Ocean

One day Mouse decided he really wanted to go see the ocean. His parents didn't think that was such a good idea; it meant a very long journey in a world full of danger. "I know what I want," said Mouse. "I've never seen the ocean, and I really want to go. Nothing is going to stop me." So his parents said, "Well, then, you'd better go—but be very careful." The next day, Mouse started his journey to the ocean. He quickly discovered what fear and danger were. A cat jumped out from behind a tree! He wanted to eat Mouse for lunch! Mouse barely escaped and ran for his life—leaving a little piece of his tail behind in the cat's mouth! In the afternoon Mouse was attacked by birds and by dogs, and he got lost several times. Poor Mouse was covered in bruises and scratches. He was tired and scared. In the evening Mouse climbed a sand dune, and for the first time ever, he saw the ocean. He watched as the waves broke on the shore. "Oh, it's so beautiful! I wish Mom and Dad were here to see this with me!" The moon and the stars came out and shone down on the ocean. Mouse was completely happy, and for a while he completely forgot his dangerous journey.

Snake and Crow

Crow was very, very hungry. He went out to look for food. When he came to a clearing in the woods, he saw a snake asleep in the sun. He jumped down on it and greedily bit it. But snakes are very supple, and some are poisonous. Snake whipped around and sunk his fangs into Crow. Crow shrieked and said, "Oh, how stupid I have been! I thought I had found a delicious meal, but now it's eating me."

Frog and Toad

Frog was swimming around in the pond after a heavy rainstorm. Up above him, a beautiful rainbow brightened the sky. Frog had heard that there was a cave filled with gold at the end of the rainbow, so he decided to go and find the cave. He swam as fast as he could for the bank. There he met Toad. "Where are you swimming in such a hurry?" asked Toad. "They say there's a cave full of gold at the end of the rainbow," answered Frog. "Come along with me, and we can share it." Frog jumped out of the pond, and together he and Toad crossed the meadow. They hopped for at least a mile before they finally arrived at the rainbow's end and saw a dark cavern in the side of the hill. "Gold!" cried Frog and Toad, and they jumped into the cave. Inside the cave lived a snake. He was hungry and had just been wondering what he should have for supper. In a single mouthful he swallowed both Frog and Toad.

Turtle and Scorpion

Turtle and Scorpion were great friends and just couldn't live without each other. One day they went out together to look for a new house. On the way they came to a river. Scorpion stood on the bank looking at the water. "Turtle, I can't swim." "Well, climb on my back," said Turtle. "I'll carry you across the river on my back, safe from all danger." Confidently, Scorpion climbed onto Turtle's back, and Turtle jumped into the water and started to swim. When they reached the middle of the river,

Turtle heard some commotion on his back. "What are you doing on my back, Scorpion?" "I am boring a hole through your shell so I can get at the nice soft flesh inside." "I thought you were my friend," yelled Turtle. "Okay then," he continued, "if you want to hurt me, I will defend myself and give you what you deserve for being ungrateful." Turtle sank down under the water and threw Scorpion off his back, then swam across the river alone. He never saw Scorpion again.

Spanky the Spider

Spanky was a very clever spider, and he wanted to become even more clever. So he set off on a journey across the world, and everywhere he went, he found clever people and animals. Spanky bought tricks from these clever people and animals. In fact, he bought all the tricks in the whole wide world! He put them in his basket and went home. When he got home, he decided to put the basket of tricks at the top of the highest cotton tree. He hung the basket on a piece of rope around his neck and began to climb. As he climbed, the basket kept banging into the tree and bonking against his stomach. Each time he got halfway up the tree, he slid back down again. Then he heard his son calling out, "Papa, why are you carrying the basket on your stomach instead of on your back like a backpack. Then you would be able to whiz up to the top of the tree!" Spanky was shocked! His son was smarter than he was. "How can that boy be so clever? I've travelled all over the world and bought smart tricks everywhere I went, yet still my son is smarter than I am!" Spanky was furious and smashed the basket to smithereens on the ground. It fell apart, and all the clever tricks flew off into the world. A couple of those clever tricks stayed with Spanky and remained with him and his children and grandchildren and great-grandchildren…all the way down to today!

Flamingo and Pelican

Flamingo invited Pelican to come and have tea. "How kind of you to invite me," said Pelican. "No one ever invites me anywhere." "I'm so glad you could come," Flamingo kindly responded. "Do you take sugar in your tea?" "Yes, please," said Pelican. When Flamingo handed him the sugar bowl, Pelican threw half the sugar in his cup and tossed the rest on the floor. "I haven't got any friends at all," complained Pelican. "Would you like milk in your tea?" asked Flamingo. "Yes, please," said Pelican. He poured a little milk in his cup and spilled the rest on the table. "No one ever comes to visit me, either," Pelican whined. "Would you like a cookie?" asked

Flamingo. "Yes, please," said Pelican. He grabbed a handful of cookies and stuffed them in his beak. His shirt was all covered in crumbs. "I would like it very much if you invited me to tea again," said Pelican. "Perhaps," said Flamingo, "but I am very busy at the moment." "Until next time, then," said Pelican. He grabbed another handful of cookies, wiped his mouth with the table cloth, and left. When Pelican had gone, Flamingo just shook his head and started cleaning up.

Peacock and Crane

One day Peacock and Crane were talking. Peacock spread out his tail and said proudly, "It's nice, huh, having a tail like this? My feathers are fit for a king, with all the colors of the rainbow and glittering with gold. Your feathers are just grey with a bit of black and white. Not really very cheerful colors." "That's true," answered Crane, "but I can fly so high in the sky that I can touch the stars, while you are strutting round on the ground like a chicken without a head." "Harrumph!" said Peacock. "You're just envious of my princely tail." "Dear Peacock," said Crane, "beautiful feathers do not make a king."

Crab and Lobster

Once upon a time, there were two very good friends, Crab and Lobster. One stormy day Crab went for a walk along the beach, where he met up with Lobster. Lobster wanted to go sailing in his boat; he just loved sailing. "Lobster, Lobster," cried Crab, "there's a storm coming, it's too dangerous!" But Lobster insisted that it was a perfect wind for sailing. "Come with me—nothing's going to happen to you." Crab thought about it for a minute and then climbed on board with Lobster. Lobster loosened the ropes and hoisted the sails, and they caught the blowing wind. The boat shot forward and sailed faster and faster until, before they knew it, they were in the middle of the ocean where the waves were as big as mountains. The wind howled and blew the boat up and down on the waves. The boat was tossed around, and the sails ripped. Crab was frightened and said, "We're going to capsize, we're going to sink!" "Hold on to me tight, here we go!" said Lobster cheerfully. Crab was scared—very, very scared. Lobster took Crab by the hand and said, "We're sea creatures, aren't we?" The boat sank, and Lobster took Crab for a walk along the sea bed. "What a wonderful adventure we are having!" said Lobster, and Crab started to feel a little better.

Owl and Duck

Owl sat up in the tree one lovely summer day. Duck stood at the base of the tree right under Owl. Duck looked up cried out, "Hey there!" "Hmm," said Owl. "Why don't you come down here?" shouted Duck. Owl yawned and flapped down to the ground. "Oh!" said Duck, "I had no idea that owls had such beautiful wings." "Hmmm," said Owl. "Why do you only say 'hmmmm'? Don't you have anything more to say?" Duck asked. "Yes, of course," said Owl, "but I am rather tired. I was asleep." "Sleeping? But it's daytime!" said Duck. "I always sleep during the day," said Owl. "How strange! Everyone sleeps at night," said Duck. "Not true," said Owl. "Night-time is far too exciting to sleep. When it gets dark, I open my eyes and ears wide and I wait till my food comes along." "You do say such silly things, Owl. Food doesn't just come along. I have to swim about and dive and search until I find something nice to eat." "Well, that sounds very strange to me," mumbled Owl. On that lovely summer day under the tree in the meadow Duck and Owl argued with each other. They just could not agree. "Duck, why are we arguing like this?" asked Owl. "Because you are always doing things wrong, that's why!" answered Duck crossly. "I'm not doing it wrong; I'm doing it differently. I do things the way owls do them." "And I do things the way ducks do them. You are right, we don't need to fight about it." "That's right," said Owl, "I am tired, and I get angry more quickly when I'm tired. Now I really need to go back to sleep, Duck." "Goodbye, Owl, sleep well." "Hmmm," said Owl sleepily, "You too, Duck, sleep well." He could hardly keep his eyes open. "Oh, sorry, you don't sleep now. You sleep when it gets dark. Have a nice day, Duck. See you again some time."

An A-to-Z on Animals and Zoos

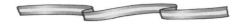

The Importance of Zoos

On a warm day it is wonderful to watch lions, apes, elephants, and hippos in the enclosures that are carefully built to imitate their natural habitats. For most children in our modern world, the zoo is the only chance they will have to hear the chilling roar of a lion, to watch tigers eating, to smell the pungent odor of rhinos, to feel the soft coat of a donkey, or to stand face-to-face with an orangutan. In the zoo you can see so many intriguing animals, some of which you will already be familiar with. But what do you really know about them? Zoos were created not only for our entertainment but also to teach us about animals from all around the world.

Today zoos also play an important role in the protection and conservation of animals. Some species now exist solely in zoos, having become extinct, usually due to a combination of factors, including humans having damaged or destroyed their natural habitats and the animal's inability to adapt to various other changes in their environment, such as climate. In the zoo, animals often behave differently than they do in the wild. For instance, an ape may take a ride on the back of a sheep and pick ticks off its back. Chimps may roll themselves up in blankets, and dolphins may swim with sea lions and play games with the trainers. Such things are possible only in a zoo, where the rules are different than the rules of nature. Animals can do anything as long as it is good for them and improves their health and well-being.

Most zoos now provide visitors with considerable information about the unique characteristics, behaviors, and natural habitats of the various types of animals exhibited there. The more you learn about different animals, the more you realize that every species is special. With that realization often comes a deeper connection with the animals and a deeper understanding of the importance of conserving their natural habitats. Their cousins in the wild often live in the most beautiful parts of the world, in the rain forests or on the plains. The species and the habitat form a whole. Zoos try to construct enclosures that are as close as possible to the animals' natural habitats. These replicated habitats help the animals to be healthier and happier while in captivity as well as to display their natural behaviors for the benefit of visitors. Their zoo homes are artificial, nonetheless, and do not negate the need to protect animals in the wild. For that reason, many zoos are trying to educate the public about the importance of conserving the natural environments of animals.

In the following pages you will find more information about the various animals you will meet during your yoga zoo adventure. They appear here in alphabetical order.

The Animals in This Book

Bears

Bears are the largest predators on dry land. Like humans, bears are *omnivorous*—which means they eat both plants and meat. They eat mostly berries, fruits, tubers, and roots as well as snails, insects, and fish. The food that brown bears love best of all is honey and the bee larvae that live in honey combs, so they put up with the bee stings. Occasionally bears hunt larger animals, such as rats and even young deer, and they sometimes eat *carrion* (dead animals). Many bears remain hidden and sleep for most of the day. Bears are incredibly strong and have long claws and sharp teeth. A bear can break the neck of a bison in one swipe, and it can crush a human to death with its strong forearms. When cornered, bears are extremely dangerous and ferociously defend their territory. If you threaten a bear, it will pull itself upright and stretch to its full height. When a bear stands upright it is considerably taller than a full-grown person. Fortunately, bears usually avoid people and rarely attack humans—except when they have young, in which case the mother bear will instinctively protect her cubs. Almost all bears are found only in the northern hemisphere. They live in forests, mountains, fields, and tundra. In the winter, they hibernate. Bears love water, and on warm days they often lie around in the water. They also have great fun with tree trunks; they sleep on them, sharpen their claws on them, float on them, roll them, and pull off the bark.

Camels

Camels can survive well in the desert because they store fat in the humps on their backs. Dromedaries have just one hump; Bactrians have two humps. Most of the camels in the world today (90 percent) are Drome-daries, and most are domesticated—which means they are raised by humans for various purposes, such as transporation, wool, leather, milk, and meat. In some places, even their dung is used as fuel! Camels are native to the deserts of Asia and the Middle East and can cope with extremes of hot and cold. Dromedaries are less able to deal with the cold. Camels grow a thick coat in the winter. The food and water they eat and drink is converted into fat and stored in the humps as emergency rations. They can go up to ten days without water and will then drink up to 32 gallons of water in one go. Camels have long eyelashes and a clear eye covering, sort of like a second eyelid, to protect their eyes from sand and dust. They are also able to close their nostrils against the sandstorms that occur regularly in the desert. The soles of their feet are very broad and have cushions, which make the feet work like snowshoes in preventing the camels from sinking into the loose sand. When camels walk they have a remarkable swaying gait that can make their riders feel "seasick." That, coupled with the fact that they can carry large loads for long distances, is why camels are known as the "ships of the desert." This swaying gait is caused by the camel moving both left feet forward (or backward) at one time and then both right feet.

Caterpillars and Butterflies

A butterfly begins life as an egg. From this egg comes a caterpillar. This caterpillar eats a lot and grows bigger and bigger. When it is big enough and fat enough, its skin starts to harden; this is called a *pupa* or *chrysalis*. Caterpillars that will become moths or butterflies spin a long thread around themselves, called a *cocoon*. Caterpillars *pupate* (change) inside this enclosure. They look as if they are dead, but they are just changing—you might say "closed for rebuilding." After a while the chrysalis bursts open, and a fully grown butterfly comes out. The wings fill up with blood and air, and then the insect sits for an hour to let them dry out before it flies away. Most butterflies fly during the day and sleep at night; most moths fly at night and sleep during the day. Wing colors and patterns provide camoflauge for both moths and butterfies.

The butterfly is one of the prettiest insects because of its large and often colorful wings. The colors and patterns on butterfly wings, just like those on moths' wings, provide protection from predators, by helping them to blend into their surroundings. So some butterflies have vividly colored and intricately patterned wings, while others have subdued colors and patterns. It often looks as though butterflies are just flying around for the fun of it, but that is not the case; they are always doing something—looking for food or for a mate. Butterflies have long rolled-up tongues with which they can suck nectar from flowers. Certain plants and trees are especially attractive to butterflies. In fact, butterflies usually lay their eggs on exactly the plant that the caterpillars will need to eat when they hatch. Safe from predators in their chrysalis or cocoon, the caterpillars will pupate and produce new butterflies or moths.

Chimpanzees

Chimpanzees are *primates* and our closest cousins in the animal kingdom. They are hairier, much stronger, and shorter than humans. They are also better climbers, but people are much more intelligent. Chimps prefer to stay on the ground. They rest and sleep in trees and make a new nest out of leaves and branches each evening. They live in groups in the jungles and plains of Central Africa, where they collect fruit, insects, and seeds and occasionally hunt. They are very inventive; for example, they use large leaves as umbrellas to keep the rain off. They also use tools, such as rocks to crack open nuts and sticks to get insects out of holes and honey out of honeycombs. Their hands are similar to human hands, which makes it possible for them to hold tools and to climb. Chimpanzees maintain strong relationships with their mothers, even when they are fully grown. An adult chimpanzee plays with her young in much the same way humans do. Their signs of affection and facial expressions are also similar to those of humans. They even use a kind of "joking face" when they want to show that they are playing and not attacking. This is to avoid getting into fights.

Chameleons

Chameleons are *reptiles*. They are covered with scales and lay eggs. They spend a lot of time sitting motionless on a branch, catching insects with a long, sticky tongue that rolls back into the mouth. The tongue is as long as the body and tail combined and functions like a kind of catapult with a sticky pad at the end. Once the prey is hit by the tongue, it sticks to the pad and is drawn back into the chameleon's mouth. This happens so swiftly that once a chameleon has spotted its prey, the bug has no escape. Chameleons have five toes that grow in groups of two and three, which act like tongs that grip firmly to branches. The long tail serves as a "fifth hand" and is rolled up when the lizard is at rest. Chameleons have no outer ear and have poor hearing. They also have no sense of smell. They can move their eyes independently of each other so they can see over a wide area. The images from the two eyes are processed in the brain to make a usable picture. They are also able to focus both eyes on the same spot, giving them stereoscopic vision and acute depth perception. This means that when a chameleon spots his prey, he can estimate the distance—which may be considerable—very accurately. Sight is therefore of utmost importance for a chameleon. As everyone knows, a chameleon can change colors, but they cannot change to any color and they don't change just to blend into their surroundings. A chameleon can display a pre-determined selection of colors and and patterns on its skin. Sometimes they do this to camoflauge themselves, but they also do it to communicate with one another (males only) and in response to temperature, light, humidity, and mood. Another weapon in their armory is their ability to puff themselves up to appear much larger so as to scare away their enemies.

Clams

Clams are *mollusks*, which are soft-bodied ocean creatures, most of which are encased in a hard shell made of calcium. There are three types of mollusks: (1) those with no shell (octopus, squid, and sea slug); (2) those with one shell (snails), and (3) those with two shells that are hinged together so they can open and close (clams, oysters, scallops). Mollusks open their shells only when they are under the water in order to eat. They filter their food out of the water. The outer rim of the shell grows as the soft body inside grows. Many mollusks live under the sand, but plenty of birds, starfish, and other predators know where to find them. Their predators eat the soft body of shelled mollucks and leave the empty shells to lie on the beach or wash in with the surf.

Crabs

Crabs come in many types and sizes, but they are all members of a branch of crustaceans called Brachyura. Like other crustaceans, crabs have an *exoskeleton* (a skeleton on the outside, rather than the inside, of their bodies) made of protein and calcium. This "suit of armor" consists of separate plates connected by thin membranes, similar to joints, so that the crabs can move. However, the exoskeleton does not grow as the crab grows, so every so often the crab *molts* (sheds) its hard exterior and grows another one. During this time, they are more vulnerable to predators. Their eyes are at the end of stalks, and they breathe through *gills*. Crabs have four pairs of walking legs and a pair of claws. Some crabs can swim very fast and others can both swim and walk well. Most can swim and walk sideways, and some can also move backward as well as forward. You will find far more empty crab shells on the beach than live crabs walking along the beach, as most hide themselves in the sand or amongst rocks, seaweed, or sea anemones. When you see an empty crab shell, you can think of it as an old coat that the crab cast aside when it got too small. If the crab was lucky, it got to grow another coat before a gull came along and ate it for lunch.

Crocodiles

Crocodiles have lived on earth since the time of the dinosaurs. When people saw the first crocodile skeletons in the Middle Ages, they thought they were dragons. Crocodiles and alligators are both members of the reptile group called Crocodilians, or "crocs" for short. Alligators usually have rounded, U-shaped snouts, and crocodiles usually have pointed, V-shaped snouts, but there are exceptions. Like all *reptiles*, crocs have scaly skin that keep their bodies from drying out and they are cold-blooded, which means they can't regulate their body temperature. So they must bask in the sun to get warm or sit under the shade to cool off. Of all the reptiles, crocs have the most complex brains and are very intelligent. They learn from experience, and use that knowledge to devise better ways of hunting. Some crocs can live for more than one hundred years. They have huge jaws with many sharp teeth, and a long tail. The eyes, nostrils, and ears are on the top of the crocodile's head. So while they are drifting under the surface of the water, they can still see, hear, and smell whatever is around—and they have very good senses. A third transparent eyelid protects their eyes in the water. They move faster in the water than on land. They swim by thrashing the tail back and forth. They do not need a lot of oxygen and can stay underwater for more than an hour. The crocodile is carnivorous and will eat any animal it can catch, but mainly it eats fish, birds, other reptiles, and small mammals. If it is able to catch a larger animal, it will do it. Crocs will swim silently to the watering holes of larger mammals; with their greenish-brown color, they are almost invisible under water. To take down a larger animal, the croc will grab the drinking beast with its teeth and drag it into the water so it drowns. Crocodiles lay eggs, usually just before the rainy season. The female croc uses her jaws to carry the young, who are able to fend for themselves after only a month.

Elephants

Elephants are the largest and heaviest land animals on earth. The elephant's most noticeable characteristic is its trunk, which is used not only for breathing and smelling, but also for picking up things, feeling around, and drinking. They also use their trunks to give things a good whack, to throw sand on their backs, and to spray themselves with water. They can even use the trunk like a snorkel, for instance, while crossing a river. Elephants live in herds consisting of females (*cows*), their offspring (*calves*), and young males (*bulls*). A daughter remains with her mother well into adulthood, sometimes for her whole life, but a son leaves the herd in his mid-teens. The males then live alone or with other immature males. All herds have a leader, or *matriarch*, which is often the oldest and most experienced female. Elephants move across great distances, and it is vital for them to know where to find food and water. They have prodigious memories, and the older elephants, in particular, will remember such things. If threatened, elephants will work together to defend themselves. The herd offers the young protection and also teaches them social skills. Though calves are a bit clumsy, they are good and determined learners and stay close to their parents. Elephants can communicate with each other over large distances through low-frequency sounds that are all but inaudible to the human ear. That is the way two herds can find each other. Wild elephants drink about 30 gallons of water a day and 220 to 440 pounds of food. They eat about half that amount in captivity, but that's still a lot! Many zoos bring the elephants' food in a wheelbarrow.

Flamingos

Flamingos have enormously long necks and legs, pink feathers, webbed feet, and curved bills. They find food by holding their bills upside down in the water, using it sort of like a fishing net. They suck water and mud into the front of their bills and then pump it out at the sides, while briny plates trap algae and shrimps like a sieve. Flamingos get their wonderful pink color from the beta carotene in their diet. Their webbed feet ensure that they do not sink down into the mud. They live in huge colonies of up to a million birds. They like brackish water in coastal marshes. Flamingo mates stay together for life. They have elaborate courtship dances, which the entire group performs together. This ensures that all the pairs produce eggs around the same time. They breed in the salt-water lakes high in the mountains and lay their eggs on mounds of mud. The chicks stay in the nest for five to twelve days, during which they are fed a type of milk that comes from the parents. Both the mom and the dad take turns feeding and looking after the young; even foster parents can feed the chicks. The chicks learn to eat and swim quickly, and when they leave the nest, they herd together in a group, called a creche.

Foxes

The fox belongs to the Canidae, or dog, family, but foxes do not live in groups like most canines. Except for when they breed and when the female is caring for her pups, foxes live and hunt alone. The fox is *carnivorous* and feeds on rabbits, birds, rodents, frogs, and eggs, but it also likes berries, nuts, and seeds. Arctic foxes also eat seaweed. In the wild, a fox marks its territory with its urine, feces, and a pungent musk excreted from anal glands. Foxes are nocturnal, doing most of their hunting at night. They generally sleep in dens made of thick brush or bushes or in hollow logs, but some foxes will sleep in the open or in trees. Foxes are mainly found in the northern hemisphere and are increasingly found in cities, although their natural habitat is woodlands and open country where they have plenty of space to roam and hide.

Frogs

Frogs are *amphibians*. They begin their lives as eggs that develop into tadpoles and then frogs. The eggs are laid in large clusters of transparent gelatinous spheres, called *frogspawn*. Some daddy frogs will carry the frogspawn on their backs to a safe place. These eggs hatch into tadpoles with tails, no legs, and gills. After a few weeks, the hind legs and then forelegs appear. Then the tail disappears and lungs form. After about three months, the tadpoles have become frogs, ready to leave the water in search of insects. Adult frogs breathe oxygen from the air into their lungs and through their skin. They have long muscular hind legs designed for leaping, pads on their toes for climbing, and smooth moist skin that easily dries out. Most frogs live in damp areas, spend a lot of time in water, and are excellent swimmers. They do not like the sun, and if there is no shadow, they dig themselves a hole and hide in the mud. The male frog can make a loud croaking sound by passing air through the larynx. That is how he calls out for a mate. The sound is amplified by vocal sacs in the throat that expand the more he croaks. The longer he croaks the louder it gets. Frogs that are a mottled brown or green color are so colored to help hide them from predators. Brightly colored hoppers, like the dart frog, are toxic; in that case, the bright color scares away predators. Some frogs also puff themselves up when a predator is near in order to make themselves appear too big to swallow.

Giraffes

At 17 to 19 feet in height, the giraffe is the tallest animal in the world. Being so tall and having 6-foot-tall necks, small heads, and long flexible tongues enable them to eat leaves from the highest trees. This is a handy feature for a plant-eater that lives on the savannah, where there are few trees and many other plant-eaters. That long neck also serves as a sort of look-out tower from which the giraffe can see predators from a long way off. Giraffes also live in herds, which is safer than living alone. Giraffes are very shy; if they hear a strange sound, they are startled and run away. They can move quite fast and can take long strides, which prevents them from stumbling over their own feet. Adult giraffes have knobs on their heads, a hump on their backs, and colored splotches all over their bodies. People sometimes say that giraffes are made of leftovers—that when animals were created, there were a few odd bits left over and that's how giraffes were made. This is nonsense, of course. The markings act as camouflage to make them harder to see amongst the trees. The small hump on their backs stores fat much like the humps on camels do. And those lumps on their heads—well, those hair-covered horns and calcium deposits seem to serve no purpose other than butting heads with one another for fun.

Gorillas

The gorilla is the largest and strongest of the *primates*, but he is a gentle giant. An adult male weighs between 300 and 500 pounds, so he is too heavy to swing from tree branches. They are 5 to 6 feet tall, and in the wild live for about 35 years. In the zoo, they can live up to 50 years. A gorilla's head is large with a low forehead and a thick, prominent brow. The palms of their hands and the soles of their feet are hairless, and their black faces are nearly hairless. Some species of gorillas have hair on their chests when young, but it disappears as they grow older. Their arms are muscular and longer than their legs. Gorillas walk upright on two feet and the knuckles of their hands; this is called *knuckle walking*, and the only primates that do it are gorillas and chimps. Their favorite foods are leaves, berries, stems, fruit, bark, seeds, and nettles. An adult male eats about 40 pounds of food a day. To drink, a gorilla dips its hand in the water and sucks the water from the hair on the back of its hand. Gorillas live in groups, called troops, led by a dominant male. A baby learns to walk at about six months but spends much of its time clinging to its mama until about eighteen months. Young gorillas continue to stay close to their mothers and share their nests until they are 5 or 6 years old. The troop moves to a different area each day, and gorillas never sleep in the same nest twice. Before each mid-day nap and at the end of every day, they make a new nest out of branches and leaves on the ground or in a tree. Generally, gorillas live at peace with each other and avoid confrontations, but if a strange male enters the group, it can lead to some elaborate behavior. This display begins with a series of screams, which get progressively louder as the dominant male becomes more angry. The high point of the show is when he pulls himself up to his full height, pulls down branches, and then beat his chest with cupped hands. He will then walk several paces toward the intruder as he growls and bares his teeth. If the stranger has not left by that time, the dominant male will attack, waving his arms wildly and shrieking angrily. The encounter generally ends with the two standing eye-to-eye and nose-to-nose until one of them finally gives up. Gorillas have no known predators, and their only enemy seems to be humans—hunters and those who destroy their natural habitats.

Ladybugs

Ladybugs are beetles, which are insects with hard bodies. Beetles come in a wide variety of shapes, sizes, and colors, but all beetles have six legs, wings, and a body made of three parts: head, *thorax* (middle section), and abdomen. The head is equipped with two eyes and two *antennae*. The legs and wings are attached to the thorax. Rigid *wing cases* cover the delicate wings to protect them. All beetles start out as eggs and go through a metamorphosis similar to that of a butterfly, changing from an egg into a *larvae* (worm), *pupa* (caterpillar), and finally a beetle. There are more than three hundred thousand types of beetles, but the ladybug is the one people like best. Beetles can be found all over the world. Most live underground, in dead wood or a dead animal, or in nests. Some beetles are plant-eaters and some are meat-eaters; some are useful to humans and some are destructive. For example, some types of beetle larvae eat wood (woodworms) and others eat roots (potato bugs). Ladybugs, though, eat bugs that are harmful to plants people eat or use for decoration in gardens.

There are actually several different kinds of ladybugs. The ladybug most people recognize is the one that is red with black spots. Many people think that the number of spots on a ladybug's back indicate its age, but that's not true. They get all their spots at the same time. Most ladybugs eat other insects. Red ladybugs with seven spots eat aphids (sometimes known as greenflies), while the yellow ladybug with twenty-one spots eats fungus.

Lions

Lions live in groups, called *prides*, with or without young, on the wide-open savannahs of Africa. Many large grazing animals live in this area, and the lion stalks them under cover of the long grass. Their sandy-colored fur makes them almost invisible on the plains. The lion is a total *carnivore*, a true hunter—but it is the females who do the hunting. One female will stalk the prey while the others distract attention by letting themselves be seen and by surrounding the animal. Then two of the lions run toward the prey, which rushes in the other direction—straight into the path of the stalker. Only when the lioness has killed her prey will the males come forward to get their share. With their big shaggy manes, the males are less suited to hunting, as they are less able to hide themselves. Many of the males live exclusively on the food caught by the lionesses. The primary role of the males is to protect the territory from other lions and to protect the pride from hyenas. Lions reserve their energy for hunting and digesting food, and they like nothing better than lying around and sleeping. Lionesses love their cubs, and, if circumstances allow, they are excellent mothers. While the cubs are still too small to fend for themselves, the mothers have to chaperone them from one hiding place to the next. By playing with each other and with the adults, the cubs learn all the tricks they need to know for survival when they are adults. The young cubs' games give them an idea of how hunting and fighting will be when they are grown.

Meerkats

Meerkats are a type of mongoose found in arid regions. They have short legs; long, thin bodies; thin fur; retractable claws; and small heads. Meerkats have a transparent membrane under the eyelid that works like a windshield when they blink their eyes and ears that close as they dig.

They also have dark bands around their eyes that reduce the glare from the sun and horizontal pupils that help them to see without moving their heads. Although their vision is excellent, they have trouble with depth perception, so they sometimes bob their heads up and down to clear their vision. Meerkats live underground in large groups of twenty to thirty, called a *mob* or a *gang*. Females are a bit larger than males. Standing on all fours, meerkats are about six inches tall; on their back legs, they're twice that tall. The mob spends a lot of time grooming, playing, and napping together. They usually go out on foraging parties—often leaving a few guards and babysitters back at the burrow—but then spread out from one another as they hunt. When one of them finds food, the others gather round, take their share, and go off alone to eat or to take food to the guards, babysitters, and young. They eat mostly insects but also lizards, scorpions, snakes, birds, and rodents. A distinctive characteristic of meerkats is their ability to eat poisonous critters without harm. Meerkats emerge from their burrows at sun-up, warm themselves and groom for a while, then forage most of the day before returning to the burrow for a good night's rest.

Owls

Owls are *birds of prey* that hunt mainly at night. They are excellent hunters, with hooked beaks, sharp claws, and two toes pointing forward and two backward on each foot, giving them an excellent grip on a branch or on their prey. Owls have exceptionally good long-distance vision. Thanks to their large eyes, they need very little light in order to see clearly. Their eyes are in the front of their heads, which helps in accurately estimating distance, but they cannot turn the eyes in the socket, so they have to turn their heads—which can in some species rotate up to 270 degrees in either direction. With their soft feathers they can fly soundlessly, which helps them to pick up the rustling sounds made by their prey. Their hearing is also very acute, with the ears hidden under the feathers on their cheeks. Owls mate for life, and both the male and female sit on the eggs and feed the chicks, which stay with their parents for three months. There are more than two hundred species of owls, and owls can be found on every continent except Antarctica.

Parrots

Tropical forests are the natural habitat for most parrots, although some live in temperate, highland, and even sub-arid zones. Parrots are easily recognized by their large heads, short neck, and strong, curved beak. The beak is very special; the upper part is moveable and is attached to the head by a hinge. The tongue is also very flexible. Although the beak appears similar to the hooked bill of a bird of prey, parrots are vegetarians and accomplished nutcrackers and seed peelers—all things they can do with ease thanks to their beaks. Many parrots are brightly colored, and they come in all sizes from very small to very large. Although they live in large groups, parrots are *monogamous*, pairing for life. They are very good at imitating sounds, which has made them very popular as pets. Some domesticated birds can even imitate human voices. They are intelligent animals, and in the wild can imitate each other and other animals. Parrots can live for a very long time—35 to 40 years. A parrot at the London Zoo lived 80 years and a wild parrot that was banded at birth in Australia lived 71 years.

Peacocks

Peacocks (male *peafowl*) and peahens belong to the family of fowl to which pheasants and chickens also belong. *Fowl* are essentially ground birds, but they can take flight when they need to. In their natural habitat, peacocks originally lived in forests and hilly terrain. Many people think peacocks are the most beautiful birds in the world. They are known for their long sweeping tails, which they can raise and open like a fan. The tail consists of about 150 beautifully colored feathers. Peahens have no tails and look very drab compared to the males. That is a good thing, because it is the female who hatches the eggs, so she needs to be as invisible as possible when sitting on the nest to avoid the attention of predators. Peacocks live in small families. A male generally has from one to five hens. Peacocks are ambulatory birds and look for food on the ground. In the early mornings and early evenings, they forage for seeds, grains, fruit, berries, insects, worms, and plants. Sometimes they pick a fly out of the air or catch a mouse on the run. Though they can run fast, peafowl are not very good at flying. They sleep in trees. At the end of the winter, they pair up. The peacock begins to get the attention of the female by calling, especially in the middle of the night. The male's call is loud and sounds like "may-awe, may-awe, may-awe." The hen answers more softly. The peacock shows off with his beautiful tail for the peahen (and also for other animals and people). At first, the female pretends not to notice, then the pair start to move around each other in a courtship dance that leads to mating. Young peafowl are born with feathers, not with down as with many other chicks. Peacocks practice their display from a very young age, vibrating their feathers and making their little tails stand up. The chicks are raised by their mothers. They ask for food by ticking on her beak and then she feeds them.

Penguins
Penguins live only in the southern hemisphere, ranging from the Antarctica to the Galapagos Islands, but excluding Australia. Most have black backs and white fronts that look like tuxedos. This coloring and pattern help camoflauge the penguin from predators, such as seals and killer whales. The penguin has wings but cannot fly. The wings have become more useful as flippers, which they use to swim. Penguins have bullet-shaped bodies that help them to swim and dive like a champ! The penguin can walk, but not very gracefully; it's more of a waddle. If they scoot along on their fronts across the ice, like a toboggan, they can go much faster. They spend most of their time in the water and come on land only to breed and to molt (shed hair). Penguins are covered with a thick layer of watertight feathers (*down*) and a thick layer of fat (*blubber*), so they won't get too cold. When they get too warm, they spread their wings open; if they get too cold, they flap their wings. Penguins do not have visible ears, just two small holes through which they hear. They see quite well, both on land and underwater, which is helpful when looking for food. They hunt fish, squid, and shellfish. Penguins make shrill cries that sound like a loud chattering. They live in large groups, staying even closer together during the breeding season. The males and females pair up to mate, but penguins that live on the South Pole cannot build a nest, because there is nothing but snow and ice. The female lays a single egg, which the male then balances on his feet. His webbed feet contain a large number of blood vessels that keep the egg warm. On the male's chest is a fold of skin that he drapes over the egg to hold it close to his stomach. The males cluster together for warmth until the *hatchlings* emerge in spring.

Rhinoceroses
Like the elephant, the rhinoceros is one of the largest and heaviest animals on earth. The rhino's most noticeable characteristic is, of course, the horn on its nose, which is made of *keratin*, the same material that human hair and nails are made of. When threatened, a rhino will charge directly toward the enemy in order to use its horn as a weapon. Even

though rhinos have big and cumbersome bodies, they are able to run fast. Rhinos love water and like to roll in the mud to cool themselves off. The layer of mud that remains on their skin afterward protects them against mosquitoes and the heat of the sun. Rhinos often have tick birds on their backs, which peck off and eat the insects and parasites on their skin. Rhinos have very poor eyesight, and at a distance of 3 feet, they can't tell the difference between a tree and a person. However, they can turn their ears in all directions, which enables them to hear what is behind as well as what is before them. They can also smell things at a distance of 925 yards, and they use their sensitive noses to explore new spaces. Rhinos can even recognize one another by each other's distinctive odor. Rhinos make a variety of sounds, including snorting, puffing, growling, screaming, shrieking, and grunting. There are different types of rhinos, two of which, the black rhino and the white rhino, live in Africa. The black rhino generally lives alone and eats mainly leaves, while the white rhino lives in a group and eats grass. There are additional varieties in Asia, all of which eat leaves, have armour plating, live in the forest, and are becoming increasingly rare.

Sea Lions

Sea lions are large *marine mammals* whose distinguishing characteristics include a smooth coat, tiny ears, whiskers, and soulful round eyes. They have two long flippers in front and two flippers behind with a small tail in between. They use their flippers to swim in the water and to climb and clamber on land. Sea lions have a thick layer of fat on their bodies, enabling them to swim in ice-cold water. When they swim, they "fly" through the water by flapping their flippers. They generally swim at about five miles per hour, but when hunting or being hunted they can go as fast as 25 miles per hour. Sea lions eat a variety of fish and squid. Their sensitive whiskers help them to detect movement in the water when they are hunting as well as to find their food in dark or murky water. Sea lions are mammals, so they breathe in air above the water, but they can remain for up to 15 minutes underwater, and they can dive deep—as much as 600 feet. In the wild, sea lions live in a harem, a group of up to fifteen females (*cows*) and young animals grouped around a single mature male (*bull*). The bull is the boss and protects the cows and the young. A fully grown cow weighs from 110 to 600 pounds, with the bull weighing in at a massive 440 to 2,200 pounds. A baby sea lion, called a *pup*, can find its mother among hundreds of cows by the sound she makes. Sea lions are very noisy creatures, indeed, and fill the air with barks, trumpets, roars, honks, and bleats.

Sloths

Sloths spend their time hanging upside down from trees in the South American rain forest. Sloths are not really slothful; no animals are lazy. They are simply *nocturnal* animals that move from branch to branch and tree to tree very slowly, as if in a slow motion. They almost never come down to the ground, as they can only drag themselves along. At top speed, sloths move 3 inches per minute. They spend almost their entire life hanging upside down in trees. They eat, sleep, and move upside down; they mate upside down; and they give birth to and raise their children upside down. Sloths can tilt their heads all the way back, so they don't have to see things upside down all the time. Their body is well-designed for this lifestyle. Their four feet are very long and have strong, curved claws that help with clinging and climbing. They only let go when they move to another branch. A sloth can stand upright, but rarely does, and he can barely walk; he is much better at swimming. They live from one meal to the next. Favorite foods are the leaf buds and shoots that are so plentiful in the rain forest at all times of the year. They pick the leaves with their lips and teeth rather than with their paws. There is little nourishment in leaves, so they have to eat a great deal. But even the sloth's metabolism is very slow, and they only need to defecate once a week. In order to do so, however, they have to climb all the way down to the ground. They dig a hole in the ground to use as a toilet. The sloth has two layers of fur—the first is short and supple and the other is much longer and coarser hair that points backward so that the rain will roll of its back as it hangs upside down. Sloths always have many parasites living in their fur as well as algae, which gives the fur a greenish tinge that is useful as camouflage amongst the leaves. It's also good for the insects who can feed off of the algae.

Sharks

Most people think sharks are horrible, ruthless, man-eating fish. Sharks are certainly powerful *predators*, but they do not normally hunt humans or attack them for no reason. When a shark attacks a human, it usually is a case of mistaken identity. To a shark prowling for food underwater, a person swimming along above them—especially on a surf or boogie board—looks very much like the shark's favorite meals—a sea lion, seal, or sea turtle. The most dangerous sharks to humans are the great whites, tigers, and bulls—because of their size, strength, aggressiveness, and widespread location. But other kinds of sharks are also responsible for at least one-third of all shark attacks on humans. Sharks have razor-sharp teeth, and they grow new ones continuously, as their teeth fall out and wear down. They also have large, extra-strong jaws. Large sharks, such as great whites, have rows of *serrated* teeth, and a specially designed upper jaw that dislocates from the skull and drops down, enabling the shark to open its mouth very wide. Their skin is so rough that in the past humans used it like sandpaper. Sharks are almost all muscle, and they swim by moving the tail fin back and forth. They steer and brake with the pairs of pectoral and pelvic fins. They are not able to swim backward, as they cannot use the pectoral fins like pedals. The dorsal fins help them to maintain balance. Most sharks move constantly, because they will sink if they stop swimming, as they do not have the gas-filled swim bladders to keep them afloat that other fish have. Sharks have six senses that help them when hunting. With their acute sense of smell, they can smell a single drop of blood in a huge tank of water. They can see and focus even better than humans, and a special tissue behind their eyes reflects light back to the retina, helping them to see well in dark or murky water. Though sharks have no visible ears, they hear very well. Their sixth sense, which comes from a lateral line along their body, allows them to detect and read *electromagnetic waves*. Sharks use *electrosensory* to navigate by the earth's magnetic field and to locate prey by their electrical impulses.

Snakes

Snakes are *reptiles*. Reptiles are cold-blooded, meaning they are not able to keep their body temperature sufficiently high without some external source of heat or cool without moving to a cooler place. Snakes are found in most parts of the world, including the oceans. In the wild they can bask in the sun or get warmth from the ground. Reptiles are not found in the polar regions, as it is far too cold there. Snakes are recognizable by their long, slender, flexible bodies and by their lack of limbs, feet, hands, outer ears, and eyelids. Their bodies are covered with strong, watertight *scales*. Snakes are *carnivores*, which means they hunt and eat other animals, particularly rodents. They cannot chew their food and so swallow their prey whole. They have *forked tongues* with which they smell and taste; they even use their tongues to detect the warmth of prey. They cannot hear in the normal sense, as they have no outer or inner ear, but they are very sensitive to vibrations, which they can feel through their bodies. Snakes can be roughly divided into two types: constrictors and poisonous snakes. They kill their prey either by crushing them to death with their powerful muscles or by poisoning them with a bite to paralyze or kill them before they swallow them. Unlike other reptiles, snakes shed their skin in one piece. Most snakes regularly cast their skins when new scales have formed underneath.

Spiders

Spiders are not insects; they are *arachnids*. Spiders have two body parts and eight legs, while insects have three body parts and six legs. A spider's body consists of a hard front part and a soft abdomen connected by a narrow waist. They usually have eight eyes and two *antennae* (feelers). Spiders are fluid feeders; they do not eat their prey by swallowing them. Instead, they spit out or inject a digestive substance that dissolves the insect so they can suck it in. Spiders have no ears, but they detect sound as vibrations through the hairs on their feet. Spiders are famous for their webs. The silk with which they spin webs is very strong and comes out of spinnerets at the back of the body. The web acts as a net to catch and immobilize insects. Some webs are sticky to prevent the insect from escaping. The silk threads also serve as a rope with which the spider can climb back up to safety if it gets knocked off. The female is usually larger than the male, mainly because she has to carry a large number of eggs in her body. Some females even carry the babies around in a protective sac for a while after they've hatched. Spiders live alone; a female will seek the company of a male only when she wants to mate. Some females eat the male once they have mated, not to be vicious but because the proteins in the male spider are important for the development of the offspring. All spiders are *carnivorous* (meat-eaters), and many are *venomous* (poisonous), but most are harmless to humans. Only a few spiders have venom that is toxic to people, and very few have venom that is potentially fatal to people. Spiders are actually quite useful. They eat a lot of insects and thus preserve the balance of nature. Without spiders, there would be far too many bugs and that would have a detrimental effect on plant life that is food for other animals, including humans.

Starfish

Starfish (or sea stars) live on the ocean's floor and belong to the group called *echinoderms,* which includes sea urchins and sea cucumbers. There are many different types of starfish, most of which have five arms, but they can have up to fifty. All starfish are predators, and they search for food constantly. Sometimes they are so hungry that they swallow their prey, shell and all. Even other starfish aren't safe! On the underside of the arms are hundreds of tiny tubular feet that work like a hydraulic system and suction cups to enable starfish to move and to capture and hold onto prey. Then all they have to do is to pry open the shell with their strong arms, push out their stomachs, and engulf the soft animal inside. If a starfish loses an arm it simply grows a new one. Starfish can move in all directions and move all their arms up in every direction. When not hunting, eating, or mating, they hide in the sand or cling to rocks.

Tigers

Tigers belong to the *feline,* or cat, family. All tigers have striped fur, which helps to camouflage them amongst the foliage. There are six subspecies of tigers, with colors ranging from varying shades of orange to tan, black, and white. Thanks to the soft pads under their feet, tigers can stalk prey without being heard. A tiger is immensely strong, and its body is built in such a way that it can catch and kill very large prey, such as water buffalo. Just as with domestic cats, the tiger can withdraw the claws on its forepaws. The hind legs are longer than the front legs, making it possible for the tiger to make huge leaps. In daylight they cannot see as well as humans, but in the dark their vision is six times better. Tigers have excellent hearing and can clearly hear each other growl at a distance of more than a mile away. A tiger is a solitary animal with its own territory. Although they live and usually hunt alone, they will frequently share the larger prey they have killed with other tigers. The others will know from the growl if they are welcome to join the feast or not. Each tiger has its own distinctive scent. A tiger will patrol the borders of its territory so that other tigers will know by the smell that one is living there. They also make scratch marks on the trees with their claws. They prefer to live in areas thick with vegetation, and most tigers love water. In the tropics, in particular, they love to play and swim in the water, like children at a swimming pool. Female tigers are some of the sweetest and most caring mothers in the animal kingdom. For three years they care for the cubs, teaching them all they need to know about hunting and survival.

Turtles

Turtles are *reptiles,* and they belong to a species called *chelonians* that also includes tortoises and terrapins. Generally, turtles spend most of their time in water, *tortoises* live on land in arid zones, and *terrapins* spend time both on land and in water but always live near water. Chelonians (referred to as turtles from here on) have existed almost unchanged for around two hundred million years. Their most noticeable characteristic is, of course, their shell, which has an upper plate (*carapace*) and a lower plate (*plastron*). The turtle can pull its head, tail, and four feet into its shell to protect those soft body parts from predators. But the shell is part of its skeleton, so a turtle cannot leave its shell and it can feel pain and pressure through its shell, just as humans do through fingernails and toenails. Turtles are *omnivores,* like humans, which means they eat both meat and plants. They are the only reptiles that have hard edges along their mouths (which look sort of like beaks) instead of teeth. They can't move their tongues much, so they are messy eaters. Some turtles return to the beach where they were born to lay eggs. Turtles make nests in sand, soil, or vegetation. Some species lay only a few oblong eggs while others lay dozens to one hundred or more round eggs. When baby turtles hatch, they are on their own, which is why some species head straight for the safety of the ocean to escape the many birds that love to eat baby turtles. Babies emerge from the egg, after hacking their way out with a special tooth, fully formed, so most can use their hard-edged mouths to crack open and eat food immediately.

Zebras

Zebras are often found living in close proximity to giraffes, as these tall neighbors can see danger first and warn the zebra. Zebra are related to horses and donkeys, the *equid* family. They have the same body type as a horse, with a long muzzle, a mane, a long tail, and four, single-toed hooves. Zebra are easy to recognize by their black (or brown) and white stripes. Another distinguishing feature is their eyesight, which is as good at night as that of an owl. Zebras live in large herds, with smaller groups forming around a stallion. In contrast to giraffes, buffalo, and antelopes, zebra are not ruminants. They chew each mouthful of grass completely before swallowing. This is why zebra spend more time grazing than do other animals on the plains. The zebra is a very polite eater; it is content with the driest and hardest grass that the other animals won't touch. Zebras spend most of the day grazing, and when there is little food around, they will continue searching at night. Most herds are nomadic and move from place to place in search of food. Zebras are very social and communicate with one another with facial expressions, including a wide-toothed "smile," and with sounds that include braying (like a donkey), barking, snorting, and snuffling (blowing out nostrils). If you see two zebras gently biting one another, don't worry; these peace-loving creatures aren't fighting, they're just grooming one another.

Games with Special Requirements

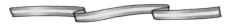

SmartFun *activity books encourage imagination, social interaction, and self-expression in children. Games are organized by the skills they develop, and simple icons indicate appropriate age levels, times of play, and group size. Most games are noncompetitive and require no special training. The series is widely used in schools, homes, and summer camps.*

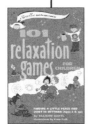

101 RELAXATION GAMES FOR CHILDREN: Finding a Little Peace and Quiet In Between *by Allison Bartl*

The perfect antidote for unfocused and fidgety young children, these games help to maintain or restore order, refocus children's attention, and break up classroom routine. Most games are short and can be used as refreshers or treats. They lower noise levels in the classroom and help to make learning fun. **Ages 6 and up.**

>> 128 pages ... 96 illus. ... Paperback $14.95 ... Spiral bound $19.95

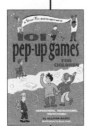

101 PEP-UP GAMES FOR CHILDREN: Refreshing, Recharging, Refocusing *by Allison Bartl*

Children get re-energized with these games! Designed for groups of mixed-age kids, the games require little or no preparation or props, with easier games toward the beginning and more advanced ones toward the end. All games are designed to help children release pent-up energy by getting them moving. **Ages 6–10.**

>> 128 pages ... 86 illus. ... Paperback $14.95 ... Spiral bound $19.95

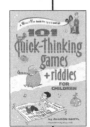

101 QUICK-THINKING GAMES + RIDDLES FOR CHILDREN
by Allison Bartl

The 101 games and 65 riddles in this book will engage and delight students and bring fun into the classroom. All the games, puzzles, and riddles work with numbers and words, logic and reasoning, concentration and memory. Children use their thinking and math and verbal skills while they sing, clap, race, and read aloud. Certain games also allow kids to share their knowledge of songs, fairytales, and famous people. **Ages 6–10.**

>> 144 pages ... 95 illus. ... Paperback $14.95 ... Spiral bound $19.95

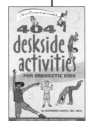

404 DESKSIDE ACTIVITIES FOR ENERGETIC KIDS
by Barbara Davis, MS, MFA

This movement resource book is written for pre-K–3 teachers, especially those who have ADHD mainstreamed children in their class. The small movement breaks can be used to keep a consistent energy and attention level in the students and go from activities for developing gross motor skills, pre-reading shapes, and alphabet recognition to progressively more complex skills and concepts. Helpful illustrations clarify many of the activities. **Ages 3–9.**

>> 176 pages ... 95 illus. ... Paperback $14.95 ... Spiral bound $ 19.95

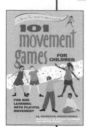

101 MOVEMENT GAMES FOR CHILDREN: Fun and Learning with Playful Movement *by Huberta Wiertsema*

Movement games help children develop sensory awareness and use movement for self-expression. The book features reaction games, cooperation games, and expression games, and some old favorites such as Duck, Duck, Goose as well as new games such as Mirroring, Equal Pacing, and Moving Joints. **Ages 6 and up.**

>> 160 pages ... 49 illus. ... Paperback $14.95 ... Spiral bound $19.95

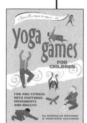

YOGA GAMES FOR CHILDREN: Fun and Fitness with Postures, Movements and Breath

by Danielle Bersma and Marjoke Visscher

A playful introduction to yoga, these games help young people develop body awareness, physical strength, and flexibility. The 54 activities are variations on traditional yoga exercises, clearly illustrated. Ideal for warm-ups and relaxing time-outs. **Ages 6–12.**

>> 160 pages ... 57 illus. ... Paperback $14.95 ... Spiral bound $19.95

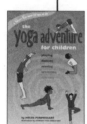

THE YOGA ADVENTURE FOR CHILDREN: Playing, Dancing, Moving, Breathing, Relaxing *by Helen Purperhart*

Offers an opportunity for the whole family to laugh, play, and have fun together. This book explains yoga stretches and postures as well as the philosophy behind yoga. The exercises are good for a child's mental and physical development, and also improve concentration and self-esteem. **Ages 4–12.**

>> 144 pages ... 75 illus. ... Paperback $14.95 ... Spiral bound $19.95

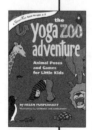

THE YOGA ZOO ADVENTURE: Animal Poses and Games for Little Kids *by Helen Purperhart*

Little children go on a journey of discovery through a zoo. Every activity of the day, from brushing their teeth to meeting all kinds of strange and wonderful animals, is accompanied by a yoga stretch, exercise, or idea as the kids come face to face with a tiger, look in the eyes of a giraffe, or waddle like a penguin. A combination of exercise, learning, and creativity in one handy package. **Ages 3–7.**

>> 144 pages ... 49 illus. ... Paperback $14.95 ... Spiral bound $19.95

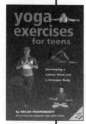

YOGA EXERCISES FOR TEENS: Developing a Calmer Mind and a Stronger Body *by Helen Purperhart*

This book can help teens to improve their physical and mental health and self-image. The exercises, divided into static postures, dynamic postures, and exercises in pairs, help reduce stress and increase body awareness. The dynamic and partner exercises aid physical development and can be used by the whole family. **Ages 13–18.**

>> 160 pages ... 62 illus. ... Paperback $14.95 ... Spiral bound $19.95